AF334401

Communication & Information Management in Radiology

ahra

Table of Contents

Acknowledgments

This project to produce the second book in the AHRA professional development series was no light undertaking. With a topic of communication and information management in radiology, it had to address a very wide scope of material and at the same time meet the rigorous standard set the by the first book in the series—*Financial Management in Radiology*. Without the commitment of the 16 AHRA member authors and 13 AHRA member reviewers this would not have been possible. We greatly appreciate the sponsorship of Bayer HealthCare Pharmaceuticals for their very generous educational grant that makes this series of books possible. In addition to the AHRA authors and reviewers, we could not have been successful without the dedication of the AHRA staff that orchestrated the management of the project, including Debra Murphy, Kathy Delaney, and Selene Steneck. Lynne Dodson proved a tremendous asset to this book with her editing, writing, and critique of literary styles to make sure the writing of the book was consistent. We also thank ITC for the typesetting and layout. And, lastly, we acknowledge Ed Cronin for his oversight, support, and liaison with Bayer HealthCare Pharmaceuticals during the progression of the project.

Patricia Kroken, FACMPE, CRA
Ellie Richardson, RT(R), MDIV
Wayne Stockburger, JD, MBA, RT(R), FAHRA, FACHE

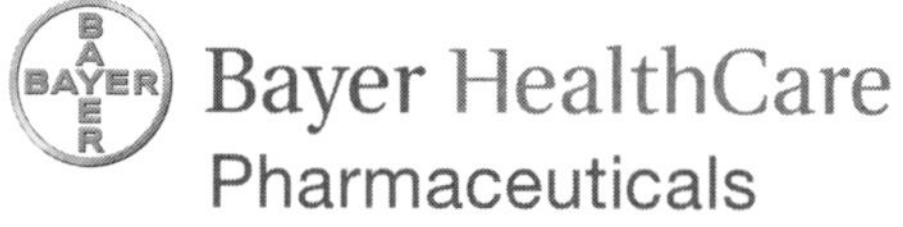

Introduction

When the Certified Radiology Administrator (CRA) program was proposed to the attendees of the 2002 AHRA Annual Meeting, no one could have imagined the success the program would have achieved in its first 5 years with over 600 imaging management professionals credentialed. In the development of the CRA program it became apparent that while there was a clear and distinct body of knowledge common to radiology administrators, there were no seminal references that contained this body of knowledge to which aspiring radiology administrators could turn to for answers to common questions, for research for personal and career growth, or for knowledge to better qualify them for the job at hand. To this end, the leadership of the AHRA commissioned the first in a series of textbooks to provide for this need. The first in the series, *Financial Management in Radiology*, has set a very high standard of quality to which this second book and all subsequent ones must adhere. The authors of the financial book consolidated a vast amount of knowledge and practice common to radiology administrators into a single text that could be used by imaging professioanls irrespective of their experience, education, or capabilities. It proved successful for the task in which it was developed.

The authors of this second book, *Communication & Information Management in Radiology*, represent the diversity in imaging management and represent all components of the industry from academic, private, and community hospital based imaging departments, multi-facility healthcare system imaging departments, imaging centers, and free standing imaging practices. This book addresses a wide variety of questions associated with the practice of information management in radiology and the communication of information within radiology and between radiology and the medical community in which it resides. Many imaging facilities and departments have begun the transition to electronic image information management, but not all. Some are further along the path to completion, but nearly all are at different places on the road to the information super highway in electronic image information management than everyone else. None have shared all the same experiences, and none have had total success without some amount of pain. While this book will not be an antidote for pain, it does endeavor to provide a framework for understanding of the needs and opportunities associated with transition from analog to electronic communication and information management in radiology.

In Part 1, Strategic Planning, there is discussion of performing a baseline analysis, identifying goals, quality improvement, resource identification, strategy development, definition of success, and communication of results.

In Part 2, Internal and External Communications, chapters review methods of communication for imaging from print though electronic, marketing, and face-to-face communication.

In Part 3, Applying Technology, the content explores information technology, image and digital data management, and the organization of information.

The establishment of the AHRA Leadership Institute, announced at the 2006 AHRA Annual Meeting as a result of the collaborative efforts of some of the visionary leaders in our industry, further promotes educational development with the need for greater educational opportunities for all of our membership, which this book endeavors to augment and support. As the industry evolves, it is crucial that radiology administrators grow with the changes around them. Without an understanding of the electronic components of information management, that change is made more difficult, if not impossible. *Communication & Information Management in Radiology* is an important tool for the radiology administrator, and will prove to be a valuable resource as the information revolution continues.

Patricia Kroken, FACMPE, CRA
Ellie Richardson, RT(R), MDIV
Wayne Stockburger, JD, MBA, RT(R), FAHRA, FACHE

Editors

Patricia Kroken, FACMPE, CRA
Vice President
Healthcare Resource Providers
Albuquerque, NM
Pat Kroken is one of the principals in Healthcare Resource Providers, a radiology business consulting firm located in Albuquerque. She is a former radiology practice manager and HRP currently works with radiology groups, imaging centers, hospitals, billing companies, and billing software vendors from coast to coast. Ms Kroken is a Fellow in the American College of Medical Practice Executives, a CRA, and a frequent speaker and author on radiology management topics.

Ellie Richardson, MDiv
Executive Director
North Shore Magnetic Imaging Center, Inc (NSMIC),
and North Shore P.E.T. Imaging, LLC (NSPET)
Peabody, Massachusetts
Ellie Richardson has been executive director at NSMIC for 19 years and at NSPET for 2½ years. She has more than 30 years' experience in imaging education and administration in both community hospital and free-standing settings. Ms Richardson holds a master of divinity degree from Andover Newton Theological School in Newton, MA, and is a graduate of Northeastern University's radiologic technology program in Boston.

Wayne Stockburger, JD, MBA, BSRT, FAHRA, FACHE
Assistant Executive Director
Scott and White Health Systems
Temple, Texas
Wayne Stockburger is administrator of the departments of radiology, radiation oncology, and orthopaedics for Scott and White Health Systems in Temple, TX. He has had many years of experience in the practice of radiology, clinically as a technologist and administratively in academic and community hospital settings.

Mr Stockburger holds an MBA from the Anderson School of Management at the University of New Mexico, and a JD from Northwestern California University School of Law. He is an active member of the AHRA, American College of

Healthcare Executives, and American College of Medical Practice Executives with fellowships in the AHRA and ACHE.

Editor/Writer

J. Lynne Dodson

Creative Lines
Stratford, Connecticut
J. Lynne Dodson, a medical writer and editor since 1971, specializes in practice management, healthcare administration, patient education, and medical history. She is the author/co-author of 7 health-related books for general audiences, most recently, *Hot Times*, ghostwritten for bestselling nutritionist Ann Louise Gittleman, PhD. Ms Dodson is also the author of 5 photographic histories of medicine and a contributing author to the *Journal of Oncology Practice*. She has twice won writing excellence awards from the American Medical Writers Association. Through her Stratford, CT based business, Creative Lines, she also provides public relations services to nonprofit organizations.

Contributors

Robert P. Brice BSRT(N), ARRT, CNMT
Director of Radiology
St Mary's Regional Medical Center
Enid, Oklahoma
Robert P. Brice is currently the director of radiology at St Mary's Regional Medical Center. He is a 1982 graduate of Marymount College of Kansas with a bachelor of science degree in pre-med (biology) and is a 1983 graduate of Wesley Medical Center Nuclear Medicine Technology School in Wichita, KS. He was team leader in nuclear medicine, CT, and MRI at Integris Bass Baptist Hospital in Enid, OK, and director of radiology at Enid Regional Hospital at the time of its closure. He has been published in *Financial Management in Radiology*. Mr Brice is married with 5 children and resides in Enid.

Deniese M. Chaney, MPH
Senior Manager
Healthcare Practice
Accenture LLP
Efland, North Carolina
Deniese Chaney is a senior manager in the Healthcare Practice with Accenture LLP. She has been associated with consulting organizations since 1998, performing operational design, operational strategy, operational transformation, and information technology engagements in provider organizations since that time. For 25 years, before entering consulting, she was at the University of North Carolina at Chapel Hill and UNC Hospitals (now UNC HealthCare). Ms Chaney held management positions in the School of Medicine as the administrative director of ophthalmology and the administrative director of radiology, and at UNC Hospitals she was director of radiology.

While at UNC, Ms Chaney was active in regional and national management organizations and was the regional president of the Eastern Region of the Radiology Business Managers Association. While at UNC Hospitals, she was co-chair of the Imaging Council of the University Health System Consortium (UHC) and national committee chair for the development of the UHC PACS Business Guide.

Ms Chaney holds a BAS in business education from Elon College in Elon, NC, and a master of public health degree in health policy and administration from the UNC School of Public Health. A North Carolina native, Ms Chaney lives in Efland, NC, with her husband, Ed. She enjoys fitness activities, gardening, fishing at the river, and time at home with family when not traveling.

Angela Colbert
Chief Executive Officer
Grapevine Imaging and Pain Management Center
Grapevine, Texas

Angela Colbert is chief executive officer of a thriving outpatient diagnostic imaging center. She holds a master of business administration degree in healthcare management with a bachelor of science degree in healthcare administration. She is a frequent speaker on healthcare issues and a consultant for radiology and pain management practices. Ms Colbert is an active member of the AHRA, Radiology Business Management Association, and American College of Healthcare Executives.

Gary L. Duehring, PhD, CRA, RT, FAHRA
Administrator
Avant Imaging Centers
Southeastern Michigan

Gary L. Duehring received his undergraduate degree from the University of Michigan, his master's degree from Central Michigan University, and his doctorate from Columbia Southern University in Alabama. He actively participates within the profession as a member of the AHRA and the American Society of Radiologic Technologists. Dr Duehring became a Fellow of the AHRA in 2006 and currently serves as a commissioner for the Radiologic Administrators Credentialing Commission.

Roberta M. Edge, MHA, CRA, FAHRA
Director of Imaging Services
Sutter Gould Medical Foundation
Modesto, California

Roberta "Robbie" Edge is the director of imaging services for Sutter Gould Medical Foundation. She has more than 20 years of experience leading imaging services in a variety of settings, from large level II trauma hospitals to a multispecialty physician clinic.

Ms Edge holds a master's degree in health administration from Chapman University in Orange, CA, and a bachelor's degree in general psychology from

California State University, Northridge. She also has a certificate in radiologic technology from Lankenau Hospital in Philadelphia.

One of the inaugural certified radiology administrators, Ms Edge also has Fellow status in the AHRA, is a past president of AHRA, and was the recipient of the Gold Award in 2006. She was also given a GE Healthcare Award for Excellence in 2006. She has authored numerous articles in *Radiology Management* and *Link*, as well as chapters in some of the other books in this series. Ms Edge is a frequent speaker at AHRA conferences. In her spare time, she is an amateur cyclist, a gardener, and an avid reader.

Maureen R. Firth, MS, RT(R)(M)(QM)

Assistant Director–Radiology and Imaging
Hospital for Special Surgery
New York, New York
Maureen R. Firth is the assistant director, North Division, of radiology and imaging at the Hospital for Special Surgery. She is an active member of the AHRA and has many years of experience in radiology. Ms Firth holds a master of science degree in radiologic and imaging sciences from Thomas Jefferson University in Philadelphia and a bachelor's degree in healthcare management from Madonna University in Livonia, MI.

David Fox, MBA, CRA

Administrative Director of Radiology
Baptist Health System
Little Rock, Arkansas
David Fox graduated from the University of Central Arkansas in Conway with a bachelor of science degree before completing his nuclear medicine technology training at Baptist School of Allied Health in Little Rock, AK. Mr Fox holds a master of business administration degree from Oklahoma City University. He is an active member of the AHRA, American College of Healthcare Executives, Society of Nuclear Medicine, and Radiology Business Management Association and is a certified radiology administrator.

Patti Hoehn, BS

Administrative Assistant
Baptist Health Medical Center–LR
Little Rock, Arkansas
Patti Hoehn received her bachelor's degree from Great Plains Baptist College in Sioux Falls, SD, and has many years of experience as an administrative assistant in the healthcare, legal, real estate, government, and financial industries.

Luis O. Marquez, MBA, MPH, FAHRA, CRA, R(R)(CT)

Director, Imaging Services

Doctors Hospital

Dallas, Texas

Luis O. Marquez is the administrative director for imaging services at Doctors Hospital. Mr Marquez received a bachelor of science degree from Fort Hays State University in Hays, KS, a master of public health degree from Wichita State University, and a master of business administration degree from Regis University in Denver, CO. He is an active member of the AHRA and the American Society of Radiologic Technologists, as well as a certified radiology administrator.

Elsa Ozuna-Richards, MSA, CMPE, ARDMS

Founder and President

REA Healthcare Strategies

Reno, Nevada

Elsa Ozuna-Richards' healthcare career has spanned many facets of the medical arena. With more than 20 years of experience in healthcare, Ms Ozuna-Richards developed strong skills in combining the clinical side of healthcare with the competitive business aspect of the industry. Her specialties include practice management, financial management, project development, A/R management, and marketing and public relations. She brings hands-on practical knowledge of the clinical setting gained as a diagnostic medical sonographer and radiologic technologist.

Her understanding of clinical operations and workflow, in combination with her expertise in developing strategic marketing goals for organizations, establishes the foundation for teaching her peers how to conduct effective market research and develop strategic plans for the medical facility. She holds that it is critical to know one's own customers/patients, their needs, and their service expectations, as well as to have solid market research as a foundation for developing strategic growth.

Ms Ozuna-Richards received her bachelor of arts degree in public administration and master of science degree in administration–healthcare management. She now heads REA Healthcare Strategies, a healthcare research and consulting firm. REA Healthcare Strategies conducts market research to drive strategic growth for healthcare businesses.

Dorothy Peare, BA, RT(R)(M), CRA

Director of Diagnostic Imaging
Community Hospital of Ottawa
Ottawa, Illinois

Dorothy Peare is the director of diagnostic imaging and women's services at Community Hospital of Ottawa. She has 17 years of leadership experience in operations; management; staff recruitment and supervision; budgeting; policy and procedure development; corporate compliance; quality improvement; and federal, state, and accreditation regulations. She received her bachelor's degree in business administration from Lewis University in Romeoville, IL, and is working on a master of business administration degree. Ms Peare became a certified radiology administrator in August 2004, is registered in radiography and mammography, and has a license from the Illinois Emergency Management Agency.

Kimlyn N. Queen, MSM, CRA, RT(R), CT, MR

Director of Imaging Service
Marion General Hospital
Marion, Ohio

Kimlyn N. (Sorrell) Queen is the director of imaging services at Marion General Hospital. She received a bachelor's degree in business administration and a master of science management from Mount Vernon Nazarene University in Columbus, OH; she is a certified radiology administrator. She received the distinguished honor of Manager of the Year for 2006 from Marion General Hospital. Ms Queen has 18 years of experience in radiology, 7 of which have been in radiology management.

Adrian Riggs, MBA, CRA, RT(R)(CT)(CV)(MR)

Operations Manager
Solano Diagnostics Imaging
Fairfield, California

Adrian Riggs has 15 years of clinical experience in radiologic sciences, both technical and managerial. His imaging experience spans all modalities and includes certification in MRI, CT, and cardiovascular imaging. He holds a bachelor of science degree in physiology from California State University, Fresno, and a master of business administration degree from California State University, Sacramento. He has worked primarily in the outpatient imaging profession and has been instrumental in implementing PACS at several northern California radiology departments.

Jim Sutton CRA, FAHRA, RT

Radiology Director

Fairmont Medical Center–Mayo Health System

Fairmont, Minnesota

Jim Sutton is the director of the radiology department at Fairmont Medical Center. He has more than 30 years of experience in the radiology cardiology field, in academic, community, and for-profit settings. In addition, he has extensive experience as a consultant in the healthcare setting. Mr Sutton is an active member and Fellow of the AHRA and is a certified radiology administrator.

Mark A. Watts, BS, RTR, CRA

System Manager, Imaging

Provena Health

Joliet, Illinois

Mark A. Watts is the IT imaging leader in the 6- hospital and 24-clinic Catholic Healthcare System. He is an active member of the AHRA Education Foundation Board. Mr Watts was named one of the Top 25 Innovators in Imaging and IT for his research in IT/patient safety. He has been a certified radiology administrator since 2002.

Elisabeth Yacoback, BSRT (R)(M)(QM) ARRT, CPHQ

QA/Education Coordinator of Radiology

Baptist Health Medical Center–LR

Little Rock, Arkansas

Elisabeth Yacoback received her radiography certificate from Cambrian College of Applied Arts and Technology in Sudbury, Ontario, and her bachelor's degree from Florida Hospital College of Health Sciences in Orlando, FL. Ms Yacoback is a certified professional in healthcare quality. Her memberships include the AHRA, National Association for Healthcare Quality, and American Society of Radiologic Technology.

Ed Yoder, RT(R), MHA

Administrative Director of Medical Imaging

Medical Imaging Department

Winter Haven Hospital

Winter Haven, Florida

Ed Yoder has more than 15 years of varied imaging management experience. He received his associate of applied science degree in radiology while completing his radiology training at the Cleveland Clinic. He went on to obtain a bachelor of arts degree in psychology from Baldwin-Wallace College in Berea, OH, and then his master of hospital administration degree at St Francis University in Joliet, IL. He is an active member of the AHRA and is on the AHRA Board of Directors, the Editorial Review Board of *Radiology Management,* and the AHRA Audio Conference Design Team. He has written many articles for *Radiology Management* and has also authored chapters in other AHRA books. Mr Yoder is also involved with the Healthcare Financial Management Association and the American Society of Radiologic Technologists.

1

Strategic Planning

Chapter 1

Performing Baseline Assessments

Jim Sutton

The accuracy and value of a strategic plan depends on the available quality and quantity of information on which that plan can be based. The radiology administrator is wise to take the time to conduct baseline assessments of trends, current capacity, human resource issues, and public perception about the organization before devising a strategic plan. In many cases, the data already exist—for example, from patient volume reports—and just have to be tabulated. In other instances, special surveys or focus groups may have to be conducted or the literature searched. Analysis of the facility's strengths, weaknesses, opportunities, and threats (a SWOT analysis) can help the administrator to accurately determine goals and future plans.

Any attempt at strategic planning will be effective only if plans are based on the best information available. Conducting baseline assessments will provide valuable data from which to identify areas for improvement or expansion, secure funding and other resources, and measure success. Baseline assessments should cover (1) trends, both within the facility and beyond it to include the overall economy and healthcare industry; (2) current capacity; (3) staffing levels and other human resource issues; and (4) the perception of the facility in its market.

Establishing Trends

The ability to foresee the future is an aptitude that few people possess. Nevertheless, all radiology administrators can build a future view of the organization by closely examining historical data and public information.

Internal Trends

Facility/Department Trends—Every facility's database contains considerable data that can serve as the basis for projections and trend analysis. For example, a radiology administrator might collect and compare data for the three most recent years on the following parameters:

- *Patient volume*—the number of patients (inpatient and outpatient for hospital-based facilities) treated by month or quarter.

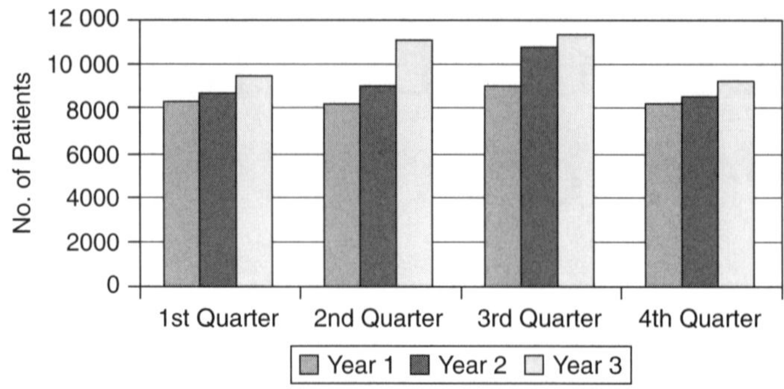

Figure 1.1 Three-year patient volume for XYZ Imaging Center.

- *Procedure volume*—the number of procedures, by modality (for example, magnetic resonance imagining [MRI] or computed tomography [CT]).
- *Patient demographics*—demographics charted by sex, age, diagnosis, zip code, or a combination.
- *Reimbursement levels*—rates per major third-party payor for key procedures.
- *Referral levels*—number of referrals occurring within a designated time period organized by referring physician or facility.
- *Capital expenditures*—amounts spent on upgrading general office equipment, imaging devices, facilities, or a combination.

Figure 1.1 and Table 1.1 present 3 years of quarterly patient volume data in alternative formats for a hypothetical facility. A review of the data reveals the following:

- The fourth quarter consistently has the lowest volume.
- Patient volume has increased every quarter of each year.
- The percentage change upward has been nearly the same for several consecutive years.

For data that are less consistent or clearcut than in the example, the analysis should attempt to identify mitigating factors—especially one-time-only events or factors

Table 1.1 Three-Year Patient Volume for XYZ Imaging Center

Year	1st Quarter	2nd Quarter	3rd Quarter	4th Quarter	Total	Variance Compared with Previous Year (%)
1	8250	8143	9000	8125	33 518	
2	8625	9000	10 744	8500	36 869	↑10
3	9400	11 024	11 250	9250	40 924	↑11

that are capable of being changed in the future. A significant decline in patient volume in the fourth quarter of the second year, for example, might be associated with office renovations that affected hours of operation. These mitigating factors should be noted in the trend analysis.

Organization/system trends—The trend analysis must move outside the facility in ever-widening "circles of influence." Hospital departments or outpatient centers (or freestanding facilities) are affected by plans and activities of the hospital administration and of other departments. Freestanding facilities, whether they are joint ventures and/or independent for profits, are influenced by decisions made by other organizations and systems in marketing, equipment, and ease of use. Radiology administrators in these facilities need to collect organization-wide data that will help provide a context for the department's data. It is useful to track the following trend data:

- *Occupancy rate.* A hospital's declining occupancy over several years is a negative trend that could signal declining inpatient referrals to the imaging department.
- *Medicaid and free care levels.* The proportion of Medicaid patients to third-party or private pay patients helps determine whether the hospital or outpatient center balances its budget and has funds available to support department needs.

The radiology administrator should collect strategic plans for other departments and for the facility overall. It may be worthwhile to hold quarterly meetings among all department administrators to exchange information on healthcare trends.

External Trends

No facility functions in a vacuum. Trend analysis should include local and state economic data and projections such as employment rates, changes in population levels, and demographics within the facility's service area, and population health data. Recent legislative changes that affect businesses or healthcare organizations should be identified. Such data are available through state or local economic development offices, health departments, and healthcare organizations.

Professional organizations and colleagues in other parts of the country can provide information on trends that eventually may affect all facilities. For example, are third-party payors piloting major changes in one region that, if successful, are likely to be implemented nationwide? What legislation is the US Congress considering that could affect healthcare? Using association listservers and chat rooms and attending meetings and conferences are ways to connect with knowledgeable colleagues. Professional publications also are useful resources for identifying trends.

No analysis of trends is complete without an examination of the future of imaging technology: "The electronic age of imaging began in the 1970's with the CT and ultrasound; has moved through digital angiography and fluoroscopy, nuclear medicine, and MRI; and is now moving into digital radiography/computed radiography (DR/CR) and mammography."[1(16)]

With digital imaging formats come ever-increasing numbers of images and more data to manage in a reproducible manner. According to consultants and industry experts, connectivity of all the modalities—the radiology information system (RIS), hospital information system (HIS), electronic medical record (EMR), and pharmaceutical venues—will be the important wave of the future. This connectivity will make the management of information and data easier and more reliable, but significant challenges must be overcome before reaching that point. Manufacturers, trade shows, professional association meetings, and colleagues are valuable resources to clarify the nature of this connectivity and how it might affect patient care within an organization.

Assessing Current Capacity

A facility's capacity depends on available technology, staffing, financial resources, workflow (see Chapter 2), and organizational structure. Organizational structure has an influence on assessing capacity. There are more or less resources available based on their philosophical convictions if they are a for profit, not for profit, joint venture, or part of a system. Analyzing each of these variables will offer a clear picture of existing capacity to meet patient needs and reveal barriers to building future capacity.

Technology Assessment

A baseline technology assessment starts with a description of existing resources and their capabilities. The assessment should be based on personal observation and research, documentation, comments by users, and accepted industry standards. The radiology administrator should do the following:

- *Describe the RIS.* Document the brand, age, and capabilities of the equipment. How well does this system integrate with other systems?
- *Describe the dictation system.* Document the brand, age, and capabilities of the equipment. Is it a digital or a voice recognition system?
- *Describe the image transmission system.* Is it adequate for department needs? Is it compliant with Digital Imaging and Communications in Medicine (DICOM) standards?

SIDEBAR: Key Elements of Technology Assessment

- Any attempt at strategic planning will be effective only if plans are based on the best information available.
- Conducting baseline assessments will provide valuable data from which to identify areas for improvement or expansion, secure funding and other resources, and measure success.
- Considerable data exist within every facility's database to serve as the basis for projection and trend analysis.
- Professional organizations and colleagues in other parts of the country can provide information on trends that eventually may affect all facilities.
- According to consultants and industry experts, connectivity of all modalities—the radiology information system (RIS), hospital information system (HIS), electronic medical record (EMR), and pharmaceutical venues—will be the important wave of the future. This connectivity will make the management of information and data easier and more reliable, but significant challenges must be overcome before reaching that point.
- Only rarely will an organization have the necessary financial resources to carry out all its goals. The budget process usually involves setting priorities, making choices, and compromising.
- Much of the information collected will also be useful in conducting a SWOT analysis. This tool, which underpins the planning process, is used to analyze an organization and its business environment.

- *Describe the scheduling and billing system.* Is it an integrated system or two separate systems? How well does the system work—for example, rate of billing errors, ease of training, and rate of double booking or other scheduling errors?

Each existing piece of equipment should be evaluated in terms of years of reliable service left, cost to operate, and volume of use (including data for the past 2 to 3 years to highlight declines or increases). User data can highlight areas of system incompatibility, inadequate or outmoded technology, workflow issues, or the need for additional training.

Financial Commitment to Capacity

Only rarely will an organization have the necessary financial resources to carry out everything it would like. The budget process usually involves setting priorities, making choices, and compromising.

Within that context, an administrator seeking to assess current capacity must review the level of financial support for staff, as well as for technology and other capital expenditures. Reviewing budget estimates in comparison with actual spending for the past 3 years can give insight into the adequacy of spending for current capacity.

Budgets that regularly fail to cover expenditures will hinder capacity growth and should be evaluated to establish the reasons for the failure to make budget and for ways to improve future budget plans. Facilities with balanced budgets may still benefit from an analysis of how expenditures are contributing to capacity and what could be done differently to expand capacity in future years.

Capital expenditures have a dramatic impact on capacity and, of course, an equally dramatic impact on a facility's bottom line. The administrator must determine if an effective process is in place to fund capital expenditures. Such a process usually incorporates a 3- to 5-year plan with a replacement budget and a mechanism to fund strategic capital investments for new, innovative equipment.

Assessing Staffing Levels and Other Issues

Given the service nature of healthcare, no baseline assessment is complete without evaluation of staffing levels, employee capabilities, and related human resource issues. Administrators in facilities with human resource departments may find that the needed data are already available; others may have to carry out surveys and records analysis to establish a worthwhile baseline.

A staffing assessment can include any of the following reviews:

- *Staffing levels.* Calculate turnover rates for administrative and direct service staff, utilization levels by type of procedure and facility (for practices with multiple sites),[2] utilization levels of temporary staff, and length of position vacancies.
- *Staffing resources.* Identify the primary sources for new staff—for example, contract agencies, direct advertising, referrals from colleagues, and affiliated hospitals.
- *Staff capabilities.* Create a skills and knowledge base assessment by reviewing current job descriptions, comparing them with the employees' actual duties, and reviewing employee performance evaluations.

Carrying out a survey of current employees and referring physicians can also help develop a baseline assessment of staffing. Using a written questionnaire or focus group, the administrator (or a consultant) can ask employees about work tasks, job satisfaction, problems related to inadequate staffing, and topics for training. The answers to these questions can provide valuable insight into staffing deficiencies. So can the answers to a brief questionnaire to referring physicians focusing on satisfaction with the facility's staff, any specific problems, and unmet needs. If the facility uses a patient satisfaction survey (see Chapter 2), the radiology administrator can review surveys from the past 12 months; identify problems related to staffing; and categorize them according to whether they are the result of process, training, or resources.

Assessing Public Perception

A patient satisfaction survey is also an effective tool for assessing how the facility and its work are perceived within its market. An administrator who believes the staff is caring and compassionate may be surprised to read patient comments such as "I was kept in the dark about what the technologist was doing" or "The staff was too busy to answer a question." A comment such as "The staff made the procedure less stressful than expected," though positive, also signals a possible misperception about the procedure that the facility may want to address.

A random telephone survey is another way to determine the public's perception of the facility. Such a survey is probably best conducted by a consultant who is experienced in devising questions that will elicit the information needed and who has a staff specially trained to effectively carry out the survey. Respondents will not necessarily be patients; they will base their responses not on actual experience but on what they have seen or read in the media or heard from friends or healthcare professionals. This broader perspective is helpful because it can reflect negative perceptions that may be causing potential patients or referring physicians to use a competing facility.

The perceptions of referring physicians should also be assessed, although they may be harder to determine than patient perceptions. Devise a *short* survey; send it with each report, including a self-addressed, stamped reply envelope; or conduct the survey in a follow-up telephone call. The survey could include three to four statements—for example, "The report was clear and informative."—to be responded to on a scale of 1 (not at all) to 5 (exactly as needed). A similar survey, with relevant statements, could be given to the staff in referring physicians' offices and hospitals.

Performing a SWOT Analysis

Carrying out trend analysis and assessing current capacity, staffing, and public perception will take time, but the effort will pay off when an administrator and others seek to devise a strategic plan, as outlined in the rest of Section 1. Much of the information collected will also be helpful in conducting a SWOT analysis, a tool that underpins the planning process.

A SWOT analysis is used to analyze an organization and its business environment.[3] A *strength* describes what the facility is good at, especially in comparison with other facilities in the region. For example, image accuracy is not a strength; it is a necessity that is expected of all facilities. In contrast, affiliation with a major teaching hospital is a strength if other facilities are unaffiliated. A *weakness* is a feature that is lacking, puts the center at a disadvantage, or both. An out-of-the-way location is usually a weakness. *Opportunities* usually refer to market conditions that the facility cannot directly control but that it may use to its advantage to increase market share. (A facility may not be able to take advantage of all opportunities identified.) A facility located in a community that is experiencing a large population growth has an opportunity to increase its patient base, for example. Finally, *threats* are external factors that may negatively affect the facility or the industry as a whole. For example, new state regulatory legislation could be a threat to net income for all facilities within the state. Strengths and weaknesses are internal factors. Opportunities and threats are primarily external factors. The following lists include additional examples that could pertain to a facility.

Strengths
- *Capabilities*—16/40/64-slice CT; 4D ultrasonography.
- *Resources or assets*—building owner; endowment designated for radiology.
- *Experience or knowledge*—staff or physician longevity; specialized training.
- *Innovation*—participation in national research trials; applications of cutting-edge technology.
- *Location*—ease of access; secure; off-street parking.
- *Accreditation or certification*—full American College of Radiology (ACR), Joint Commission, American Registry of Radiologic Technologists (ARRT), Certified Radiology Administrator (CRA) certification, subspecialty certifications.
- *Systems or communications*—exceptional patient satisfaction survey results; presence of a staff person dedicated to physician relations.

Weaknesses
- *Financial characteristics*—bad debt; low cash flow.
- *Location*—no parking; a declining neighborhood perceived as unsafe by patients.
- *Staffing*—inadequate staffing for patient load; compensation below regional standards.
- *Experience, knowledge*—high turnover rate; failure to update training.
- *Leadership, commitment*—inexperienced leadership; poor management of staff or facility.
- *Systems, communications*—lack of integration among key systems; high level of rejected third-party billing submissions.

Opportunities

- *Demographics*—major senior complex built nearby; aging of baby boomer generation.
- *New markets*—addition of physician with subspecialty certification; new satellite office.
- *Organizational*—joint ventures; merger with another for-profit facility.
- *Government/regulatory*—grandfather clause for new regulation; tax incentive for urban relocation.
- *Patient volume*—closing of a competitor; moving of additional referral sources into the community.
- *Innovation*—new procedure shown successful; development of innovative equipment by manufacturer.

Threats

- *Human resources*—tight job market for certified technologists; fewer graduates of radiology technologist programs.
- *Competition*—opening of a new facility; updating of imaging equipment by another facility.
- *Economy*—loss of major employer; pressure for lower reimbursement rates.
- *Government*—mostly new workplace regulations; formation of healthcare oversight committee.
- *Public opinion*—rise of safety concerns; changing patient needs.

This list for a SWOT analysis is by no means all-inclusive, but it provides a starting point for any administrator's own analysis. If researched properly, the SWOT analysis can be the basis of successful strategic planning.

References

1. Griffin D, Dubiel P. Thinking strategically about diagnostic imaging capacity and capital. *Radiol Manage* 2006;28(1):15–22.

2. New staff utilization survey provides data on staffing levels, FTE volume. *Radiol Manage* 2005;27(1):46–48.

3. Sferrella SM, Allen ML, Reitter MS, eds. *Financial Management in Radiology.* Sudbury, MA: American Healthcare Radiology Administrators; 2004: 247–248.

Chapter 2

Identifying Goals and Areas for Improvement

Robert P. Brice and Maureen R. Firth

A strategic plan is based on goals, and setting those goals is based in part on the identification of areas that need improvement. Goals provide a mechanism by which everyone in the organization can measure their performance. Goals also give order and direction to the workday and help the facility grow. Among the sources of worthwhile goals are work processes, internal customers, and external customers. Tools include workflow analysis, review of productivity statistics, accreditation processes, focus groups, one-on-one interviews, and surveys.

Strategic planning involves the combined efforts of many personnel to develop action steps and produce decisions to define what an organization will become. The process identifies what a facility will do, and why it will do it, to benefit others and itself. Strategic planning also identifies a facility's goals and areas in need of improvement, revision, or removal. The process involves ongoing self-assessment and analysis of work processes with the goal of positive insight and growth within an organization.

Goals provide a set of stated expectations for everyone to work toward and to give staff members a sense of order, direction, and meaning. An organization will usually have both long- and short-term goals, with the long-term goals remaining in place for a considerable time and the short-term ones subject to change. When carefully outlined, a facility's goals will specify results and outcomes that all staff will consider worth achieving. Finally, effective goals specify the quality or quantity of the desired result so that everyone will know when a goal has been achieved.

The following are some examples of strategic goals for a facility:

- Increase volume in a particular imaging modality by 8% over the previous year.
- Increase market share over a competitor by 3%.
- Increase the customer satisfaction percentage over last quarter in outpatient imaging services.

The baseline assessment outlined in Chapter 1 provides the foundation for identifying areas in need of improvement and setting worthwhile goals. In particular, any healthcare organization is likely to succeed by focusing its planning and goals on three areas: work processes, staff members and other internal customers, and patients and other external customers.

Work Processes

Conducting a Workflow Analysis

A workflow analysis is the ongoing evaluation of processes that either support or undermine the strategic vision of a department, an organization, or both. Analyzing the existing workflow helps expose the dynamics within a facility. It includes evaluating all current processes, beginning with an analysis of both internal and external work process components. The results will be broad at first but will become more defined with further analysis.

Internal Analysis—Internal assessments are part of a comprehensive review of workflow and how its processes contribute to an organization's goals for improvement. A variety of methods can be used, including the following:

- Focus groups.
- One-on-one or small-group communication.
- Indirect communication by way of methods such as surveys and suggestion boxes.

Focus groups and one-on-one communication are particularly effective in identifying broad areas of concern. Surveys are useful for revealing specific issues and details, especially because of their anonymous nature (to be discussed later). Internal assessments have the advantage of taking place within a controlled environment with controllable results, and they involve a limited and select group. A possible disadvantage is the lack of diversity in view among the participants.

The internal analysis of workflow dissects which processes work and which do not. This introspective observance of internal structure seeks to answer questions such as these:

- Are current work steps and processes an advantage or a hindrance to the strategic plan?
- Do the workable processes further the organization's strategic initiative?
- Do current processes work or need revision?
- Which productive steps are to be maintained or removed?

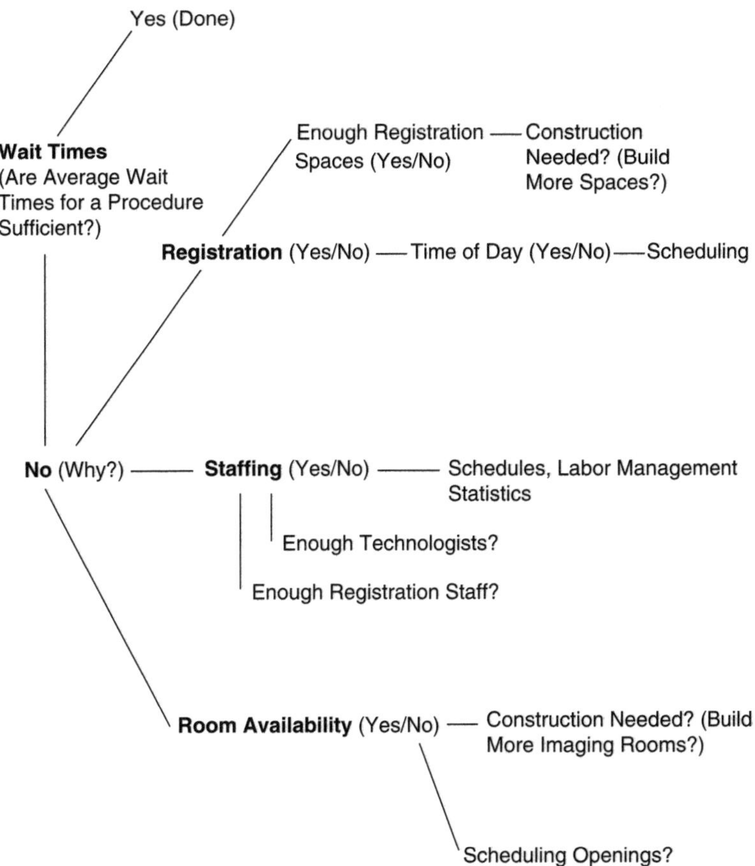

Figure 2.1 Sample process map: wait times for procedures.

A simple process map offers a visual representation of each step in a process (Figure 2.1).

External Analysis—Using focus groups for external assessment as an alternative or additional retrospective review of workflow can be as productive as an internal assessment in documenting appropriate goals. The personnel selected for this group are those individuals who are directly affected by the work processes and who have the greatest impact on the final results; they may work in ancillary departments directly related to radiology functioning (for example, laboratory, patient registration, or business office) or be more removed (for example, hospital, clinic, board of governors, or investors). Freestanding imaging centers would benefit the most from external focus groups that consist of previous clientele that have visited the facility and their physicians. The clientele could consist of vendors, visitors, patients, their families and their physicians. Their offered input for improving workflow will assist in the formulation of improvements that can be made for these facilities. The use of questionnaires, follow-up phone interviews, and direct conversation to referring physicians offers the best insight for improvements.

The benefit is a more global view of how workflow will affect the "big picture" within the organization. An external assessment is a definitive evaluation from a different vantage point. This type of focus group offers diversity and a broad view of work processes and problems, frequently giving insight to things that may have been overlooked through the use of internal assessment methods.

External analysis involves a third-party review of the current workflow processes in terms of how well work tasks contribute to the strategic plans of others and, in a hospital, to the institution as a whole. This objective review seeks to answer questions such as the following:

- Does the facility's workflow meet the expectations of others?
- Do tasks have a positive impact on the success of others, either directly (as in patient registration) or indirectly (as in the institution as a whole)?
- What external factors need to improve (for example, report turnaround, patient wait time, or patient transport)?

Analysis of Processes—The workflow analysis will identify processes that contribute positively to achieving the facility's goals—for example, a wait time of less than 15 minutes per patient or same-day mammography screening and diagnosis. The analysis is an opportunity to examine whether the positive influences that enabled accomplishment of the goals were human factors or mechanical processes. Positive influences help build a strong foundation on which to improve the organization's performance.

Equally important is to identify the negative or detrimental factors—what is not working—by asking questions such as the following:

- What has been implemented with little or no impact on workflow?
- What has had a detrimental effect that prevented meeting the desired outcomes?
- What processes that are not effective now did work in the past?

Proposing Workflow Changes—No matter how effective a facility is, potential improvements in work processes will always be identified. A process that worked at one time may no longer meet the facility's needs, or patient expectations may change and existing processes no longer satisfy them. New staff members may bring experiences of best practices that could enable the facility to exceed current goals. Whatever the reason, once a process is identified for reassessment, the next step is to propose changes by way of goals. The following can help ensure success:

- Communication is critical. Affected staff should know what problem has been identified, help develop the necessary changes, and set a goal.
- Process changes must be accepted by all individuals affected to ensure consistent application and achievement of a goal.
- All changes to the work process should be clearly delineated and any training provided before changes are fully implemented.
- A visual display (for example, a flowchart) of the new process may help some staff members better understand and adopt the changes.
- Results (or lack of results) should be tracked and communicated on an ongoing basis, allowing for additional changes, training, and communication to ensure goal achievement.
- An environment that encourages constructive analysis and creative thinking will ensure that processes are always challenged and new goals set.

When changes are proposed, measurable goals should be established to evaluate the success or failure of the changes and, if necessary, to make the case for additional changes. Constant evaluation of measurable goals will lead to refinement of tasks in order to support the success of the organization's goals and improvement within its strategic plan. For example, if the process for checking in patients is to be changed, a standard for wait time per patient should be set, based on best practices and industry guidelines. Measurement is a simple process of logging time of entry in registration, time of check-in to the imaging department, time in the procedure room, and time of exit. The results are easily quantifiable, measurable, and visual.

Compare the result to the goal. If the goal is not met, work with staff to identify problems, make additional changes, measure again, and post results until the goal is met or exceeded. Every proposed change, revision, or refinement of workflow should have a measurable result to show success or failure. These measures are the continuing effort to fortify an organization's vision, strategic plan, or both. Chapter 6 explores a number of tools to measure performance.

Measuring Productivity

According to *Webster's Third New International Dictionary*, any effort is productive if it is "effective in bringing about . . . the satisfaction of wants or the creation of utilities."[1] Unintended results usually can be traced to failure to define the "wants" to be satisfied or the "utilities" to be created.[2]

Souza et al have outlined four characteristics of productivity that contribute to its usefulness in planning and goal setting. First, productivity is a management philosophy, not a tool or statistic. It is an ongoing effort to make the most of a facility's efficiency and effectiveness. As such, it must be regularly reviewed to identify issues affecting efficiency. Second, productivity is a dynamic, relative process, not a static condition. Comparisons should be made to all facets of a facility's operations, previous internal performance, and operational goals. Third, productivity is multidimensional and should mirror the organization's primary workflow or processes. Attempts to improve patient care delivery should cut across departmental lines, similar to how a patient moves through the facility. Finally, productivity is the means to a strategic end. It means working smarter, not harder. Productivity management involves better allocation of resources to achieve well-defined operational objectives as efficiently and effectively as possible. Institutions should take the time to identify underused, unused, or misapplied resources and reallocate them to maximize overall effectiveness.[2]

An effective productivity measurement process will have the following qualities:[3]

1. *Performance.* Comparative performance should be measured in business terms against some planned activity, level, event, or standard.
2. *Quantitative.* Objective criteria should be discrete and measurable.
3. *Accountability.* Specific individuals or groups responsible for the performance should be not only identified and charged with that responsibility but also given the resources and authority to affect the performance.
4. *Auditability.* The reporting system to support the process should be consistent and supported by detailed information to show validity if the processes are ever audited or scrutinized. Do the processes work efficiently?
5. *Simplicity.* All good ideas can be presented on a single sheet of paper.
6. *Comprehensive.* The management reporting process should be complete in scope and reflect the organization's actual activities. This effort begins with the establishment of a comprehensive productivity reporting system that focuses on agreed-upon metrics. Such a system essentially manages expectations and perceptions.

Labor Management Statistics—Productivity management involves better allocation of resources, the most important of which is people. Healthcare as an industry devotes approximately 60% of its costs to labor. A fine balance between costs and staffing levels must be maintained to ensure the delivery of quality care. Changes, revisions, additions, and deletions in labor management strategies must be justifiable and sound to produce favorable results.

When used as a means to justify staffing levels to support an institution's efficiency or effectiveness, labor management statistics can be a valuable and valid tool. More accurate forecasting of staffing needs compared with projected volumes and better use of labor can lead to improved productivity and profitability. An understanding of financial labor management statistics evolves from an evaluation of a facility's labor productivity standards. These standards are usually set by the business and accounting department based on industry standards or a thorough evaluation of other facilities within the same or similar system offering the same services and product volumes.

Simple methods can be applied to evaluate the efficiency of labor management productivity and thus identify areas that may need improvement. For example, an evaluation of the total number of worked hours allowable per specific timeframe (daily, weekly, bi-weekly, per pay period, and so on) versus hours actually worked can be carried out. The result will provide the percentage a facility or service line is over or under projections. The ideal labor and productivity goal is 100% productivity, which at times is difficult to attain.

The fact that a standard for productivity per service line has been established, of course, does not mean the standard cannot be revisited and reviewed; in fact, an ongoing evaluation of the standard should be incorporated into management processes. Services must be maintained with appropriate staffing levels to ensure the integrity of patient care and of the service line without compromising patient satisfaction or safety. If the staffing level is inadequate to maintain quality services, it must be readdressed.

Maintaining the level of staffing in line with the labor management statistics is integral to ensuring budgetary compliance, but it should not hinder the growth or success of the strategic plan. To justify altering an established productivity standard, the radiology administrator should gather the following data:

- Current staffing levels in relation to peak volumes, with special attention given to inadequacies and changes in volume or workflow.
- New services to be added or deleted that will affect staffing needs.
- Changes in referral trends, such as new referring physicians, hospitals, or other healthcare facilities in the community.
- Statistical trending of volumes based on specific timeframes (such as quarterly or annually).

Using a sound justification with quantifiable data can help validate points to increase the Labor Management Statistic (LMS) standard. Remember to explain

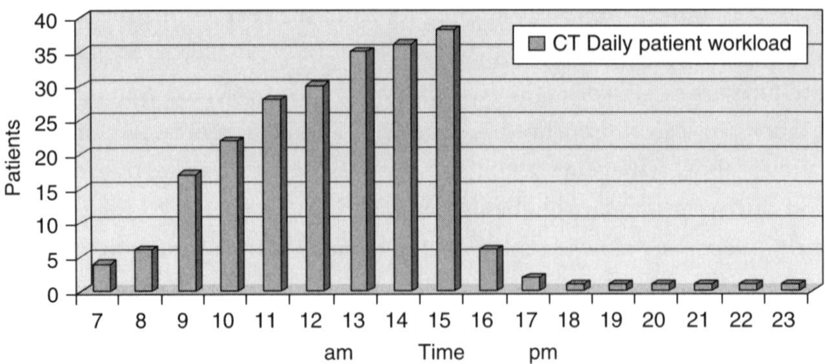

Figure 2.2 Patient workload.

how these changes will fortify the strategic plan, the organization's goals, and areas in need of improvement.

Peaks and Valleys of Productivity—An important variable of productivity that must be reviewed daily is the worked labor hours versus the work load. A day's peaks and valleys can be tracked by a postmortem review using a patient log-in sheet, modality schedule/work list, or current available radiology management software. The evaluation will readily highlight current peaks and valleys in a worked schedule (Figure 2.2). The data can also be easily quantified and presented as a bar graph or line chart for a visual representation that can be presented to staff or administration.

The same data sources can also reveal the labor hours required to provide a service per an episodic patient event. The resultant number of worked hours (regulated by the standards) should be at or above the 100% mark, provided the service is performed in a timely manner and as proficiently as possible. If the number falls out of an acceptable range, details should be provided related to mitigating factors, such as "waiting on lab, physician." How well peaks and valleys of productivity can be managed is a key indicator of whether current labor productivity standards are sufficient for staffing efficiencies. Underestimated staff coverage will tend to increase overtime or callback hours, which can be detrimental to productivity. Scrutinizing workflow provides data to justify additional staffing or staff reductions in relation to the set standards and the allowable staff levels.

An Excel spreadsheet is another mechanism by which to evaluate productivity daily and cumulatively (Figure 2.3). Not only does the spreadsheet help highlight areas in need of improvement with regard to productivity and staffing; it also serves as a useful communication tool to discuss potential changes with staff and management.

Department Productivity Report

Pay Period: 1

Department:	WIC			Cost Center:	7558/670									
Statistic	Procedures													
	Variable	Fixed												
Standard	0.77828		2 Fixed; Prod Hrs per Stat	1.32253										

		A	B	A × B = C	D	C + D = E	F	G	F + G = H	H − E = I	J	K	H + K = L	M	N	O
Day	Date	Statistic	VMHS	Variable Productive Hours Allowed	Fixed Hours Allowed	Total Productive Hours Allowed	Actual Productive Hours	Actual Agency & Contract Hours	Actual Total Productive Hours	Allowed vs. Actual Variance	Cumulative Variance	Actual Total Non-Productive Hours	Total Paid Hours	Daily Prod. FTEs	Daily Prod. %	PPTD Prod. %
Sunday	12/26/2004			0.00		0.00			0	0.00	0.00		0	0.00	0.0%	0.0%
Monday	12/27/2004	35	0.77828	27.24	14.44	41.68	43		43	(1.32)	(1.32)		43	5.38	96.9%	96.9%
Tuesday	12/28/2004	30	0.77828	23.35	14.44	37.79	40		40	(2.21)	(3.53)		40	5.00	94.5%	95.8%
Wednesday	12/29/2004	35	0.77828	27.24	14.44	41.68	40		40	1.68	(1.84)		40	5.00	104.2%	98.5%
Thursday	12/30/2004	40	0.77828	31.13	14.44	45.57	43		43	2.57	0.73		43	5.38	106.0%	100.4%
Friday	12/31/2004	35	0.77828	27.24	14.44	41.68	39		39	2.68	3.41		39	4.88	106.9%	101.7%
Saturday	1/1/2005			0.00		0.00			0	0.00	3.41		0	0.00	0.0%	101.7%
1st Week Ttl.		175	3.8914	136.20	72.22	208.41	205	0	205	3.41		0	205	5.13	101.7%	
Sunday	1/2/2005			0.00		0.00			0	0.00	3.41		0	0.00	0.0%	101.7%
Monday	1/3/2005	36	0.77828	28.02	14.44	42.46	45		45	(2.54)	0.88		45	5.63	94.4%	100.4%
Tuesday	1/4/2005	40	0.77828	31.13	14.44	45.57	44		44	1.57	2.45		44	5.50	103.6%	100.8%
Wednesday	1/5/2005	35	0.77828	27.24	14.44	41.68	40		40	1.68	4.13		40	5.00	104.2%	101.2%
Thursday	1/6/2005	34	0.77828	26.46	14.44	40.90	43		43	(2.10)	2.04		43	5.38	95.1%	100.5%
Friday	1/7/2005	33	0.77828	25.68	14.44	40.13	45		45	(4.87)	(2.84)		45	5.63	89.2%	99.3%
Saturday	1/8/2005			0.00		0.00			0	0.00	(2.84)		0	0.00	0.0%	99.3%
2nd Week Ttl.		178	3.8914	138.53	72.22	210.75	217	0	217	(6.25)		0	217	5.43	97.1%	
Pay Period Ttl.		353	7.7828	274.73	144.43	419.16	422	0	422	(2.84)	(2.84)	0	422.00	5.28	99.3%	

Total Productive FTEs: 5.275   Total Paid FTEs: 5.275   Productivity Percent 99.3%

Comments:

____

____

Key: A = Stats for that day (eg, visits, procedures, and patients). B = Variable man-hour per stat (VMHS) listed as a variable component of the standard. C = Variable productive hours allowed: A × B = C. D = Fixed hours allowed per the standard per the formula:

$$\text{Hours per week} \times \text{Fixed component/Days of week service offered} = \frac{40(2)/5}{\text{Nonproductive \%}(1.1078)} = 14.44.$$ (This example was 5 days per week; if 7 days per week, enter 7 in place of 5.)

E = C + D (total productive hours allowed). F = Actual cumulative productive hours (actual payroll hours), all employees. G = Actual agency and contract hours (if any). H = F + G (Actual productive hours + Actual agency and contract). I = H − E. If H is larger, the facility is not as productive as it should be and has used more worked hours than allowed per volume. J = Cumulative variance from the level of productivity expected (I day 1 [Monday] + I day 2 [Tuesday] and so on). K= Any miscellaneous paid hours (PTO (Paid Time Off), vacation, sick , jury duty, etc). On time sheets this is the difference between paid hours and productive hours. Entering data in this field is optional. L = Same as H. M = H/8 (hours of operation); daily productive FTEs. N = E/H × 100 (daily productivity %; *should be 100% daily or by week's end and pay period end*). O = Per pay period to date productivity %:

day 1 (Monday) will be $\frac{E}{F}$; day 2 (Tuesday) will be $\frac{E\ (\text{day 1 + day 2})}{F\ (\text{day 1 + day 2})}$; and so on.

Figure 2.3 Department productivity report.

Determining Regulatory and Accreditation Compliance

For radiology administrators seeking to identify areas of improvement and to set goals for the unit's strategic plan, compliance with regulatory and accrediting standards presents valuable opportunities. Compliance with standards ensures that the facility is serious about the validity of its services and generates credibility within the community.

The Joint Commission—The Joint Commission (www.jointcommission.org) is an independent, not-for-profit organization that evaluates and accredits nearly 15,000 healthcare organizations and programs in the United States. It is the predominant standards-setting and accrediting body in healthcare. Since 1951, The Joint Commission has maintained state-of-the-art standards that focus on improving the quality and safety of care provided by healthcare organizations. The Joint Commission's comprehensive accreditation process evaluates an organization's compliance with these standards and other accreditation requirements. The mission of The Joint Commission is to continuously improve the safety and quality of care provided to the public.[4]

Accreditation by The Joint Commission is recognized nationwide as a symbol of quality that reflects the commitment of an organization to meeting certain performance standards. For an organization to earn and maintain its Joint Commission accreditation, it must undergo an on-site survey every 3 years. These surveys are unannounced, so organizations must be prepared for the next *patient*, not the next *survey*. Successful accreditation belongs to organizations that can change the cultural practices of their staff members. Unannounced surveys focus on operational systems and patient care processes. Organizations can use the accreditation process as an operational management tool. The unannounced survey presents a clear picture of daily operations and is viewed as more credible with outside organizations and the public.[5]

The Joint Commission's 2007 National Patient Safety Goals (NPSGs) promote specific improvement in patient safety. All organizations must show compliance. A score of less than 100% will result in a requirement for improvement. The scoring guidelines are as follows: 2 = compliant, 1 = partially compliant, and 0 = noncompliant.[6] Areas of concern for a facility include age-specific competencies, credentialing of licensed practitioners, information management, performance improvement versus quality control, process design, continuity of care, and data collection. The Joint Commission's 2007 NPSGs are described in the following subsections.

Improving the Accuracy of Patient Identification—Use two patient identifiers whenever providing treatment or procedures; administering medications or blood products; or taking blood samples or specimens for clinical testing. *Ask patients to spell their last name or give their date of birth.*

Improving the Effectiveness of Communication among Caregivers—When communicating verbal or telephone orders or reporting critical test results by telephone, verify the complete order or test result with a "read-back and verify" from the person who received the telephone call. *Do not leave messages on voice mail, as doing so provides no documentation that a person received the result.* Review the policy and procedures concerning which staff members may accept verbal orders and the procedure for documentation. Are they clearly stated and followed?

Standardize a list of abbreviations, acronyms, and symbols that are *not* to be used throughout the organization. Generate a list of acceptable abbreviations, acronyms, and symbols, and communicate them to the staff. *Be careful of look-alike and sound-alike medications.*

Measure and assess the timeliness of reporting critical test results and critical values. Take corrective action if necessary. *Define and measure critical values as a facility. The RIS may already have a reporting mechanism for critical values. How will this information be used for performance improvement?*

Implement a standardized "hand-off" procedure. Two clinical people are needed to communicate relevant information and to ask and respond to relevant questions required to provide appropriate care to the patient.

Improving the Safety of Medication Use—Identify and review sound-alike and look-alike drugs used in the organization. Label all medications. Label every filled medication container used in a procedure setting (for example, syringes, medicine cups, and basins). *Information that is necessary on containers may include name of medication, dosage, amount, date, and time of filling.*

Accurately and Completely Reconcile Medications across the Continuum of Care—Implement and document a complete list of medications used by a patient upon admission. Compare the medications the organization provides with the medications on the patient's list. *Instruct patients to bring all medications with them to the radiology facility, especially patients having interventional procedures. Cardiac catheterization is a primary example of the need for medication reconciliation.* Communicate a complete list of the patient's medication to the next provider of service when the patient is transferred within or outside the organization.

Other Universal Protocols for Imaging Facilities—To ensure accuracy and improve the safety of radiological procedures other universal protocols should be followed when imaging patients.

1. Verify all procedures being performed. *Make sure there are procedures related to how that information is obtained from the patient.*
2. Mark all sites for laterality. *Markers are critical for all images, especially with digital imaging equipment. Annotations on images are inserted after processing. They can be deleted as easily as they were inserted. Permanent (before processing) markers are essential for legal identification.*
3. For all high-risk procedures, take a *time out* before beginning. *Remember, the time out is the same in the operating room as in the radiology facility.*

American College of Radiology (ACR)—The ACR (www.acr.org) is the nation's leading organization of radiology professionals, representing more than 30,000 radiologists, radiation oncologists, medical physicists, nuclear medicine physicians, interventional radiologists, and medical researchers. The mission of the ACR is to serve patients and the public by advancing the science of radiology, improving the quality of patient care, providing continuing education for radiology and allied health professionals, and conducting research for the future of radiology. The ACR has established nationally recognized accreditation programs since 1966. It has accreditation programs in the following modalities: mammography, radiation oncology, breast ultrasonography, CT, MRI, nuclear medicine and positron emission tomography (PET), stereotactic breast biopsy, and ultrasonography. Accreditation programs under development include MRI breast, MRI cardiac, MRI musculoskeletal, and CT cardiac. A more flexible whole-body MRI program is under development as well.

Value of ACR Accreditation—Why should a facility seek ACR accreditation? The number one reason is quality. The ACR gives a peer-reviewed, education-focused evaluation of a practice and may document the need for new equipment. ACR accreditation also instills patient and payor confidence. ACR accreditation means certain formal reviews of a facility's services meet the criteria of state or federal government needed for some third-party payors, which affects reimbursement. ACR accreditation can also be used as a marketing tool to bring in new customers. Today many patients search the Internet to find acceptable healthcare facilities. An ACR accreditation is widely recognized as a standard of excellence. *Reimbursement is a critical point when discussing accreditation. A facility may be penalized if no accreditation is forthcoming.*

Physician Peer-Review Program Requirements—All facilities applying for ACR accreditation or renewing their accreditation must have a physician peer review program in place. RADPEER (a simple, cost-effective ACR process that allows peer review to be performed during the routine interpretation of current images) or an equivalent review program will be required for accreditation. Excluded are programs in the following:

- Mammography.
- Stereotactic breast biopsy.
- Ultrasonographically guided breast biopsy.
- Breast ultrasonography.

Examinations should be systematically reviewed and evaluated as part of the overall quality improvement program at the facility. Monitoring should include evaluation of the accuracy of interpretation and the appropriateness of the examination. Complications and adverse events or activities having the potential for sentinel events should be monitored, analyzed and reported, and periodically reviewed to identify opportunities to improve patient care. These data should be collected in a manner that complies with regulatory peer review procedures to ensure the confidentiality of the peer review process.[7]

During interpretation of a new examination, if prior images of the same area of interest exist, the interpreting radiologist will typically form an opinion of the previous interpretation while interpreting the new study. If the opinion of the previous interpretation is scored, a peer review event has occurred. In RADPEER, the reviewer scores the report of the previous interpretation using a standardized 4-point rating scale.

An acceptable alternative physician peer review program must include the following:

- A peer review process that includes a double reading assessment (two MDs interpreting the same study).
- A peer review process that allows for random selection of studies to be reviewed on a regularly scheduled basis.
- Examinations and procedures representative of the work of each physician's specialty.
- Reviewer assessment of the agreement of the original report with subsequent review (or with surgical or pathology findings).

- A classification of peer review findings with regard to level of quality concerns (that is, a 4-point scoring scale).
- Policies and procedures for action to be taken on significantly discrepant peer-review findings for purposes of achieving quality outcomes improvement.
- Summary statistics and comparisons generated for each physician by modality.
- Summary data for each facility by modality.

For information on RADPEER or e RADPEER please refer to the ACR Web site. ACR New Accreditation Physician Peer-Review Requirements are available here, as well.

Mammography Quality Standards Act (MQSA)—In 1992, through its Center for Devices and Radiological Health, the Food and Drug Administration (FDA) began enforcing the MQSA (www.fda.gov/cdrh/mammography), which regulates all facilities performing mammography. Congress passed the MQSA to ensure that mammography performed at facilities is safe and reliable—that high-quality mammography is being performed for early breast cancer detection. Early detection can lead to early treatment and increased survival rates.

Standards relate to quality assurance, staff qualifications, reports and record keeping, and other key functions. The regulatory process includes periodic review of clinical images, an annual on-site survey by a medical physicist, and an annual on-site inspection. Under this law, mammography facilities must be MQSA certified as meeting strict quality standards. Mammography facilities are inspected annually by the FDA to ensure that standards of care are being followed by technologists, interpreting physicians, and imaging equipment. Every 3 years the ACR will accredit a facility if it meets further extensive review of equipment, record keeping (including timely result reporting to referring physicians and patients), physician interpretation, and patient standards of care. Patients should look for the display of the MQSA certificate in each mammography facility that can by law perform mammography. All certificates have an expiration date, and each facility must renew its certificate before expiration to maintain regulatory FDA compliance.

American Registry of Radiologic Technologists (ARRT)—The ARRT (www.arrt.org) certifies technologists working in medical imaging, interventional procedures, and radiation therapy with a written examination and requirements for continuing education to meet annual recertification. It also certifies radiologist assistants through a review of training, clinical experience, and written case reports. ARRT certification by a facility is usually mandatory, but most states use the ARRT examination results in making licensing determinations. Technologists should show compliance to this regulatory group by passing the ARRT examination pertaining to their specific education (for example, CT, nuclear medicine, or radiography) or be registry eligible by passing an accredited school program that teaches radiology sciences.

Health Insurance Portability and Accountability Act of 1998 (HIPAA)—As a result of HIPPA (www.hhs.gov/ocr/hipaa), the Office of Civil Rights of the Department of Health and Human Services has developed standards related to patient privacy and information security that must be met by all healthcare providers. Facilities must have documented policies and procedures defining how the integrity of patient records will be maintained. An overview of HIPAA is available at www.cms.hhs.gov/HIPAAGenInfo.

State and Local Laws—Every state and local government regulates businesses within its jurisdiction, but considerable variation in regulations specific to imaging centers or radiology departments exists. Laws may relate, for example, to certification and/or licensing of staff and equipment; record keeping; financial reporting, billing, and other accounting issues; and building codes.

The penalties for noncompliance with any of the standards, regulations, and laws vary from a warning letter to closure. Fines may be levied, as in the case of HIPAA noncompliance. But noncompliance is also an invaluable educational experience and can provide meaningful goals. Some ways to use compliance or noncompliance to reveal areas for improvement follow:

1. Administrators in facilities that are already accredited should review the results of previous site visits, focusing on areas that the survey team identified as noncompliant or compliant but less than ideal.
2. If the facility has not yet applied for accreditation, the application (available online) and materials available from The Joint Commission or the ACR should be reviewed, with a focus on areas that might not meet standards. A mock review can highlight areas for improvement.
3. The FDA Centers for Devices and Radiological Health produces a scorecard that allows facilities offering mammography to compare their own results with aggregate data from other US centers. Results that fall below those of comparable facilities could signal areas on which to focus strategic planning efforts.
4. Standards and laws change from time to time, especially as evidence-based medicine documents more effective practices and procedures. Notification of revised standards is a signal to review existing practices and possibly set goals to make changes to ensure future compliance.

Internal Customers

Internal customers include the facility's staff and radiologists. For radiology facilities within a hospital or other multiservice organization, internal customers also include ancillary departments with whom the facilities interact—for example, the medical records department, the operating room, or the emergency department. Given the people-centric nature of radiologic services, these internal customers play a significant role in identifying areas for improvement and setting appropriate goals.

Identifying Concerns of Staff Members

As mentioned earlier, among the tools effective in eliciting staff input are focus groups, one-on-one communication, and indirect communication such as surveys.

Internal Focus Groups—Focus groups provide input through discussion of a specific topic and usually involve groups of 4 to 12 people. The group's composition is selected to represent individuals affected by the topic to facilitate the gathering of subjective input and opinions. The procedure involves the use of a skilled moderator—often a consultant—to ask specific questions in a permissive environment where points of view are not judged and consensus or decisions are not sought. The participants should feel free to discuss the topic. Results of the discussion should be documented (for example, taped, captured on a flip chart, or recorded in minutes or a summary report). In general, focus groups

- Involve people.
- Are conducted in a series of meetings.
- Involve participants who are reasonably homogeneous; they can be familiar with one another or be from vastly different areas of expertise for more diverse viewpoints.
- Use data collection procedures.
- Make use of qualitative data.
- Have a focused discussion.[8]

As a tool for generating ideas and information to develop a strategic plan, focus groups have the following advantages:

- The process is socially oriented.
- The moderator can probe responses for additional details.
- Members' decisions show validity.
- The cost for conducting groups may be lower than some alterative information-gathering tools.

- The timeframe from initial set-up to final information gathering is relatively short.
- Multiple groups offer larger sample sizes than do other qualitative techniques such as one-on-one interviews.

Disadvantages of focus groups include the following:

- When compared with individual interviews, focus groups have less control over the information gathered.
- Data analysis is difficult.
- Moderators need high levels of training and skill.
- Groups can vary considerably in the caliber of response, communication skills, and understanding of issues being explored.
- Groups are difficult to assemble.
- Discussion must be conducted in an environment conducive to conversation.

One-on-One Interviews—One-on-one interviews with individual employees can be time-consuming, but they can also elicit information that may not be discovered using focus groups or written surveys. Face-to-face talks have the benefit of nonverbal communication, which can offer insight into issues affecting morale, resistance to change, and staff retention. The conversations may also identify misinformation or misconceptions that could become the focus of one or more departmental goals.

Another advantage of one-on-one interviews is that they probably are already part of the organization's procedures. For example, employee performance reviews, exit interviews, and even "lunch with the CEO" events can provide valuable insight into areas that need reworking or from which goals can be set.

Although a performance review focuses on an individual employee and his or her goals, it nevertheless can be an opportunity to gather information relevant to the facility's goal setting. For example, an employee may cite deficiencies in processes or equipment that have negatively affected performance or caused significant job stress. The review may reveal low morale as a factor in the employee's performance; careful probing could bring out working conditions that may be affecting other staff members as well and that should be addressed.

Exit interviews are conducted with employees just before they leave employment and can provide a retrospective review of the facility's operations and processes. These interviews can help a radiology administrator gain insight into areas for improvement, reevaluation, and revitalization of work processes. Criticism is beneficial if it brings about changes to improve processes. Good exit interviews should also yield useful information to assess and improve all aspects of the working environment, culture, processes and systems, management, and employee development—in fact, anything that determines the quality of the organization in terms of its relationships with its staff, customers, suppliers, third parties, and the general public.[9]

A conclusive interview process can provide insight and direction toward implementation of changes to fortify an organization's goals, offer areas of improvement, and support the strategic plan. These improvements redefine directions to support enduring strategic planning or strengthen final strategic plan objectives.

In larger organizations, exit interviews may be conducted by human resources staff. In that case, a process should be in place to ensure that comments are reported to the radiology administrator for review.

Employee Opinion Surveys—Employee opinion surveys offer another valuable internal tool to guide an organization's goal setting and strategic planning. Surveys gather data anonymously by way of a series of questions on key areas such as employee functions and working conditions, department policy and practices, and the organization's administrative foundation.

David Chaudron, a consultant and author on organizational change and strategic planning, suggests the following tips to increase the effectiveness of employee surveys:[10]

- Make the survey part of the planning cycle. Schedule it early enough in the annual budget and planning cycle to effectively use the results in setting goals.
- Communicate clearly to all staff members the plans for the survey and how the data will be used.
- Keep survey data anonymous, but communicate fully about actions that are desired as a result of the data.
- Know how the data will be analyzed before administering the survey. Consider administering a preliminary survey to a representative sample of employees, and analyze the limited data. Revise questions if they seem confusing or if the analysis is too difficult.
- Consider conducting surveys several times a year to a sample of employees instead of once a year to all employees. This strategy will elicit more representative data that are less influenced by a one-time-only issue.
- Use several types of surveys; that is, send a sampling of employees an open-ended questionnaire calling for written answers and send other employees a

numerical questionnaire that simply requires circling the appropriate number. Numerical surveys are simple to complete and score, but they don't elicit many details. "Essay" surveys take more time for the respondent to complete, conceivably lowering the response rate, and they are more difficult to score.

- Involve key employees in devising, administering, and analyzing the survey and in developing recommendations based on results. These employees should be staff members who are formally or informally considered powerful by their co-workers.
- Always provide feedback and take action after a survey. Use the results to set goals. If the survey raises issues that cannot be immediately dealt with or that are out of the organization's control (for example, issues that involve legal requirements), employees should be told.
- Create a valid and reliable survey. Asking several questions in different ways on a given topic will help establish validity. Reliability relates to consistency over time, allowing comparison of results from one survey to the next.

Technology makes it relatively simple to set up online questionnaires through a facility's intranet, which can be scored electronically. However, paper surveys are flexible in terms of when and where employees can complete them; are available to employees who don't have regular access to a facility computer, such as maintenance workers; and may be considered more anonymous by staff than an electronic document.

Identifying Concerns of Radiologists

The radiologists who work for or own an imaging center have insight as to how the facility can be profitable and have a vested interest in producing professional revenue. They also share common values and culture with referring physicians and those working in ancillary departments of a hospital, such as the emergency department; thus, they may be able to present ideas from the perspective of these other groups. The physicians' concerns often relate to work processes to make workflow more efficient (scheduling, paperwork, image retrieval and review, and risk management) or to capital expenditures (technology advancement). Physicians' needs most likely will be the factors that increase speed and task turnaround times.

In addition, radiologists are valuable resources to identify issues involving quality assurance. In accredited facilities, quality assurance goals or measures will already be in place as part of the compliance process (discussed previously); many other facilities are likely to have at least some standards set as well. These results are usually measured quarterly. Evaluating the results at the end of each term will give insight to other measures in need of improvement. Setting a standard of measure that must be met each time will easily identify those areas that need less attention and others that must be quickly addressed. A quantifiable measure of an organization's expectations and results will bring about changes in steps and operations that will improve work tasks.

Quality assurance goals are usually expressed as a percentage that must be met to be acceptable. Measures continually meeting 100% can be set aside. Measures that fall short must be addressed and results gathered, measured, and reported again. Results can be shown in graphic form (for example, in charts or bar graphs) or statistically as straight percentages in tables. A person who sees a "report card" of the measurable results will take more responsibility for them, especially if the results are benchmarked against those of peers, other departments, or other facilities. What better way to strengthen an organization's strategic plan than to offer indicators that measure successes, failures, and improvements!

It is crucial to identify areas of concern to radiologists, but it may not always be easy. The process is aided by enlisting the support of the lead physician. The tools used to elicit information from staff members—that is, focus groups, one-on-one interviews, and surveys—can be used with radiologists but will need to be concise for fast completion. Regularly scheduled management and quality assurance meetings may be an opportunity to solicit information on a given topic. Reviewing error reports is one way to identify areas for improvement. The more the process of data gathering can be incorporated into existing processes, the greater the likelihood it will be carried out. As with information from staff members, feedback and communication about the goals and areas of change that arise from radiologists' information are essential for continued participation in quality assurance measures that will bring successful changes.

Identifying Concerns of Ancillary Departments

In a hospital or other multiservice healthcare organization, the imaging department must interact directly and inclusively with other departments that are also working toward optimal changes for better performance. Strategic initiatives must bring about changes that are beneficial for the whole facility.

The operation of a radiology department can be viewed in its simplest form as meeting three "wants":

1. A referring physician wants to be able to schedule a patient when needed.
2. A patient wants to "get in and get out."
3. The physician and patient want the results immediately, if not sooner.

Satisfying these wants, however, calls for much more than a well-run imaging department. Only when all departments work toward common goals and with effective communication will everyone be satisfied:

1. Scheduling.
   - The scheduling department must communicate with the physician's office or ancillary departments such as the operating room.
   - The scheduling department must communicate with the imaging department and vice versa.
   - The imaging department may need to communicate with the ancillary department from which the patient is being referred.

2. "Get in and get out."
   - The referring physician or office staff must communicate the appointment to the patient.
   - Admissions must promptly register the patient.
   - Transportation within the facility must bring the patient to the imaging department promptly.
   - Radiology reception must accept the patient promptly.
   - Radiology reception must communicate with the imaging staff.
   - The staff must communicate with the patient if delays arise.

3. Immediate results.
   - The imaging staff must ensure that films are available for prompt review.
   - Transcription staff must communicate with the radiologist and vice versa.
   - Staff must communicate results to the referring physician.
   - The report must be forwarded to medical records and be maintained or retained in the radiology department.

The workflow analysis, described earlier in this chapter, will highlight many points at which the radiology department's processes intersect with those of ancillary units. Each point is a potential area for improvement or a goal-setting opportunity, based on information supplied by employees of all departments involved. Focus groups and employee surveys involving representatives from the ancillary departments may be particularly useful adjuncts to the workflow analysis. If there is a glitch in the system, it should be recognizable as workflow or survey results are evaluated. Are these points of contention being covered in the best possible manner? If not, the problem should be evaluated, the work tasks dissected, personnel addressed, and operational methods and physical limitations that hinder results discussed.

Being able to communicate about areas in need of improvement in a constructive, blameless manner is important. Any strategic initiative can be carried out faster, easier, and with greater likelihood of success if open communication is established. Setting up mechanisms to gather information from all involved, using an inclusive process to set mutually agreed on goals with measurable results, and providing feedback on results and further need for improvement will go far toward ensuring everyone's cooperation and participation in the planning process.

External Customers

External customers represent the primary market for a facility and are its reason for existence. External customers include referring physicians, patients, and the community at large. Soliciting their input can bring a unique and valuable perspective to any effort to develop a strategic plan or to any strategic initiative.

Identifying Concerns of Referring Physicians

As noted earlier, focus groups composed of key referring physicians and surveys sent to their office staff are useful mechanisms for soliciting information relative to goal setting. Achieving full participation, however, can be challenging.

A particularly effective tool applicable to this group is a "grand rounds" appointment with each key physician in his or her office. To ensure effective time management, the radiology administrator should begin by looking at referral patterns, identifying physicians with the highest number of referrals and those who should refer but do not. Physicians in both groups should be the first visited. These data should be available through the radiology management system software, the business office, or patient accounting. Subsequent visits may target new practices to the region and practices at the middle range in terms of the number of referrals each year.

The radiology administrator might consider setting aside a designated time and day each week for one or more appointments. The visit should include conversations with both the physician and staff members who interact with the facility. This visit is an opportunity to ask what can be done to rectify problems, especially with practices that are not referring patients; ask how processes might be streamlined to make their lives easier; and listen to the staff's concerns. Radiology administrators who open up viable communication pathways in this manner may find greater participation in future surveys and focus groups as well.

An alternative is to set up quarterly or semiannual breakfast or luncheon meetings for small groups of referring physicians or representatives of their staff. These meetings are less formal than focus groups and the information supplied may be less well defined, but nevertheless valuable. It will be useful to have an agenda that is communicated in advance to give participants a chance to identify areas of concern or to solicit information from co-workers who are not attending. These meetings should begin and end promptly, focus on areas of common concern, and reinforce the message that this effort is designed to contribute to the success of their practice as well as that of the imaging facility. These are information gathering sessions, not gripe session, and they should not be used to defend organization practices.

Whether a radiology administrator chooses to visit practices or hold informal meetings, each visit or meeting should be followed by a quick thank you note for the input. If problems were identified that require an immediate response, that response should be communicated. Once goals have been set or a plan put in place, feedback should be given to all who participated.

Identifying Concerns of Patients

Like referring physicians and their staffs, patients offer a unique perspective on the organization. Whereas staff members may come to accept a process as "the way it's always been done," the patient brings a fresh view, unencumbered by day-to-day routine. A number of mechanisms readily available to gather information from patients can be useful in identifying areas for improvement and helping set the department's goals.

As described earlier, focus groups can be used to collect information on a specific topic or more general impressions. Some groups may include former patients who discuss their experiences with the center, and others may be composed of individuals who have used other facilities. The guidelines given above can ensure an effective group dynamic.

Patient satisfaction surveys or exit surveys are probably the most commonly used way to gather patient opinions (Box 2.1). The survey can be in a standardized format (Gallup poll) or by way of a customized post-visit written or verbal correspondence. Every patient can be given a short questionnaire at registration (easier in outpatient or clinic settings), which is collected after the examination by way of drop boxes in the waiting room. Patients who do not want to take the time to fill out the questionnaire at the time of service can be given the option of mailing the survey from home, but few will actually do so.

Ideally, every patient would receive a survey. However, if the facility seeks to focus on a particular service line (for example, women's imaging) or a process

Box 2.1 Inpatient Questionnaire of Services

Patient Questionnaire

This feedback form is for patients who have had a radiology (CT, ultrasound, MRI, X-ray, nuclear medicine) exam with us.

Our goal in the radiology facility is to provide complete patient satisfaction. Your feedback about your experiences will help us to serve you better in the future. We would very much appreciate a few minutes of your time to complete this survey. Thank you!

Instructions: Please think only about your most recent visit.

Your name (optional):

....

Your e-mail address (if you have one):

....

What kind of exam did you have?

.... CT
.... Ultrasound
.... X-ray
.... MRI
.... Nuclear medicine
.... Other—Please enter type of exam, if known: ....

When did the exam take place?

Date, if you remember it: ....

Did the staff explain the exam to your satisfaction? (Please circle one.)

Yes, the explanation was fine.

The explanation was somewhat confusing.

I was not satisfied with the explanation.

Please rate the cleanliness and ambiance of our imaging facility's exam area. (Please circle one.)

Excellent Good Fair Mediocre Poor

Please rate your experience during this visit with any of the following staff whom you interacted. (Please circle.)

Reception Staff .... *Technical Staff* .... *Physician*

Excellent .... Excellent .... Excellent
Good .... Good .... Good
Fair .... Fair .... Fair
Mediocre .... Mediocre .... Mediocre
Poor .... Poor .... Poor

Overall, how would you rate your visit to our imaging department? (Please circle one.)

Excellent .... Good .... Fair .... Mediocre .... Poor

Feel free to add any comments about your experience and/or ways to improve our services. Thank you!

____

issue (for example, wait times), a representative sampling of patients can be sent a specialized survey with questions that directly relate to the goals being evaluated. If the budget allows, the preparation, distribution, and analysis of the survey can be outsourced to a consulting firm, as described earlier.

The Internet and e-mail have opened up new fact-finding avenues. Patients who are willing to provide their e-mail address on their registration forms can be sent a brief satisfaction survey that can be completed online and returned electronically. Particularly with younger patients who are used to corresponding at work and with friends by way of e-mail, this medium presents a fast, inexpensive, and responsive mechanism to gather data. Of course, a system must be in place to compile the results, analyze the information in terms of service strengths and weaknesses, and develop ways to turn this information into viable short- or long-range goals toward improvement (see Sidebar, p. 38).

Identifying Concerns of the Community and Others

Whether an imaging facility achieves its goals may be influenced by the community at large and various external groups not directly served by the facility. These groups include patients' family members, vendors and insurers, competitors, and community leaders. Information gathered from these sources may identify issues related to billing and accounting, workflow, community relations, patient relations, and best practices.

A patient satisfaction survey, for example, could include spaces for family members to respond; also, family members could be invited to take part in patient focus groups. A brief survey could be sent with checks to vendors, or vendors could be asked to complete a brief survey when they visit the facility. Community leaders could be invited to a semiannual breakfast or luncheon or be included in focus groups.

Staff members should be encouraged to belong to, and take part in, appropriate local organizations, including the chamber of commerce, civic groups, and healthcare

SIDEBAR: Identifying Goals and Areas for Improvement through Focus Groups

As strategic plans are developed and communicated throughout the facility, the use of focus groups adds diversity and insight to their formulation. As a tool for generating ideas and information to develop a strategic plan, focus groups have the following advantages and disadvantages.[8]

Advantages	Disadvantages
The process is socially oriented.	When compared with individual interviews, focus groups have less control over information gathered.
The moderator can probe responses for additional details.	
Members' decisions show validity.	Data analysis is difficult.
The cost of conducting groups may be lower than some alternative information-gathering tools.	Moderators need high levels of training and skill.
	Groups can vary considerably in the caliber of response, communication skills, and understanding of issues being explored.
The time line from initial set-up to final information gathering is relatively short.	
Multiple groups offer larger sample sizes than other qualitative techniques, such as one-on-one interviews.	Groups are difficult to assemble.
	Discussion must be conducted in an environment conducive to conversation.

associations. Although information gathered at meetings and by way of Listserv conversations is anecdotal and informal, it can nevertheless provide valuable clues to areas in need of improvement. Furthermore, networking among professional colleagues is one way to establish best practices and benchmarks against which to compare the imaging facility and even to learn about planning efforts of others that failed (and therefore should be avoided). By identifying colleagues who manage facilities similar in size and scope, a radiology administrator can establish a communication network for exchanging information on a range of topics, including information that might lead to goal setting. A quarterly conference call might be one vehicle for peer partners to broaden their knowledge base.

Radiology administrators who manage facilities that are components of a bigger organization have the benefit of a "corporate think tank" they can approach for information helpful in formulating the facility's goals or strategic plans. Other divisions may have strategic initiatives that were successful in their communities that can be adapted. Questionnaires may already exist; high-quality consultants for focus groups or data analysis may already have been identified.

Finally, what better way to gain insight and direction in relation to building organizational goals and strategic plans than to look at the successes and failures of competitors? The strengths and weaknesses of competing facilities are easily seen and can be used to avoid making the same mistakes. It is possible, for example, to identify what capital equipment has been added recently, what services are being promoted, and what modalities these represent, and then to compare this information to what is available in the facility. Substantial differences may signal an area for improvement. It is worthwhile to look at details such as hours of operation and special promotions, again with the intention of identifying potential goals.

Conclusion

The greatest strategic plans involve the best thoughts, ideas, feelings, and desires of their developers and combine them with an organization's mission or purpose to provide a stable foundation for growth and success in business. Using environmental opportunities, strategic planning is a process of developing and maintaining sensible and lucrative practices of an organization and its resources. It is the breakdown of the big picture into smaller elements that can be scrutinized, revised, restructured, or removed. When collectively rejoined under one vision, the strategic plan will ensure longevity and prosperity. The success of a strategic plan depends on the probing, discussion, and examination of the personnel who are directly responsible for ensuring the integrity of the plan when carried out. Everyone within the organization must be included in the plan's formulation, be willing to accept the plan, agree on its direction, and be willing to set into action steps to ensure its success. The best strategic plans are those based on strong, well thought out organizational goals that test the limits of conformity, are visionary, encompass the most services and service lines, and are beneficial to both the customers served and inevitably the organization.

Once a strategic plan is formulated it is important to adjust each facet to ensure solid implementation of the worked tasks and steps leading toward success. Accurate data collection with sound business practices and a solid implementation plan involving the right people will provide longevity in the market. Once sound business practices and people are engaged, a continual follow-through audit should be made to be sure that initiated processes are working and to identify those processes that may need refinement or change. This ongoing process evolves as the dynamics of the organization change in tandem with changing economic and social principles. Great ideas that make valid business or visionary strategic sense for a facility must include an extensive, sound plan of action. Using a plan of action built on a solid implementation of worked tasks that are continually followed through to completion will ensure that great ideas that support a strategic plan do not end in failure or stifle growth.

References

1. Gove PB (au), Merriam-Webster (ed). *Webster's Third New International Dictionary, Unabridged.* Merriam-Webster. 2002.

2. Souza MG, Vining GW, Read K. Four principles that lead to greater productivity. *Healthcare Financial Mgmt.* November 1990. Available at: http://www.findarticles.com/p/articles/mi_m3257/is_n11_v44/ai_9074872. Accessed January 26, 2006.

3. Hosseini A. Definitions of productivity as used in business, hospital, and academia: a summary. Available at: http://www.sonoma.edu/users/h/hosseini/productivity/Definition.html. Accessed January 26, 2006.

4. The Joint Commission. Available at: http://www.jointcommmission.org. Accessed September 14, 2006.

5. Hargis, PD. JCAHO accreditation, unannounced surveys: contributing to risk management and patient safety. Paper presented at: AHRA Annual Meeting; August 3, 2006; Las Vegas, NV.

6. Atkins, JM. JCAHO 2006–2007: Update for hospital imaging departments. Paper presented at: AHRA Annual Meeting; July 31, 2006; Las Vegas, NV.

7. American College of Radiology. 2005 ACR Guidelines and Technical Standards: ACR Position Statement on Quality Control and Improvement, Safety, Infection Control, and Patient Education Concerns. *J Vasc Interv Radiol* 2005; 16:149–155.

8. Williams E. Focus groups. Available at: http://www.hmi.missouri.edu/ course_materials/Executive_HSM/semesters/S2006/8450/boren/focus_groups.htm. Accessed April 23, 2007.

9. Exit interviews and knowledge transfer—tips for employees and employers, sample questions and answers. Available at: http://www.businessballs.com/exitinterviews.htm. Accessed February 27, 2006.

10. Chaudron D. Master of all you survey: planning employee surveys. Available at: http://www. organizedchange.com/survinc.htm. Accessed December 7, 2006.

Chapter 3

Basics of Quality Improvement

Dorothy Peare

This chapter discusses quality control, quality improvement (QI), and quality management and how they are interrelated with communication and information management in radiology. Quality control is the measure of quality. Quality improvement is the process of attaining a new level of performance or quality that is superior to any previous level of performance. Quality management is the process by which people are mobilized to achieve quality goals.[1] The basics of QI involves acknowledging that an error will occur and that when it does, a work environment that supports excellence will improve the processes and create a stronger, more effective healthcare system.

The National Association of Quality Assurance Professionals defines quality in healthcare as levels of excellence produced and documented in the process of patient care, based on the best knowledge available and achievable at the particular facility.[1] As radiology continues to move into the digital world, management of image data and the flow of information becomes a vital part of the facility's infrastructure.

Radiologic applications of information management include using diagnostic reporting systems, tracking utilization patterns of imaging modalities and various clinical outcomes, documenting the type of information sought by and provided to physicians, and evaluating the facility's quality standards and performance goals. This flow of information can be managed through a well-developed quality improvement (QI) plan.

The radiology administrator should be able to identify the role of the radiology department in the facility's overall interdepartmental QI and strategic plan. As QI activities progress, communication among team members, leadership, and departments—including nursing units, if applicable—is important. This chapter will explain models and tools that can guide the radiology QI team through the process. When this is accomplished, quality care is provided consistently to all patients and their families, wherever they may be in the organization.

History of Quality Improvement

QI began in the manufacturing industry in the 1940s and 1950s with the pioneers Philip Crosby, Joseph Juran, and W. Edwards Deming. Each expert brought his own approach to achieving QI.

Crosby defined the Four Absolutes of Quality Management:[2]

1. Quality is abiding by the rules.
2. The system for achieving quality is to prevent the noncompliance processes.
3. The performance standard is to expect excellence at all times.
4. The measurement of quality is the measure of noncompliance processes.

Crosby taught the importance of the relationships of quality and cost and of maintaining a level of compliance with defined specifications or standards. His work is based on the following 14 steps:

1. Management commitment
2. The QI team
3. Quality measurement
4. The cost of quality
5. Quality awareness
6. Corrective action
7. Zero defect planning
8. Supervisor training
9. Zero defects day
10. Goal setting
11. Error-cause removal
12. Recognition
13. Quality councils
14. Doing it over again

Juran's quality process has three parts: quality planning, quality control, and quality management. Quality planning involves identifying the customers and their needs, translating those needs into the industry language, and developing the product efficiently. Quality control is the evaluation of performance through measuring the actual performance according to the standard goals. Quality management encompasses the infrastructure and the project teams that carry out the process improvement.

Deming's philosophy centers on the development of quality and its continual improvement. Deming was instrumental in the rebuilding of Japan after World War II using this method. Many corporations, such as Disney, Dow, and 3M, adopted Deming's philosophy in their total quality management systems. Deming developed 14 principles of management, which are applied to radiology administration in the Sidebar below.[3]

The healthcare industry boom after World War II defined *quality* as "abundance" in healthcare. The United States was considered to have the greatest healthcare in

SIDEBAR: Applying Deming's 14 Points to Radiology

The following are Deming's 14 Points of Management, with explanations that provide an understanding of how to apply them to the radiology facility.

Point 1: Create constancy of purpose for improvement of product and service.

Constancy of purpose in radiology includes clinically appropriate diagnostic imaging and therapeutic radiology orders based on a patient's past history and current disease process; an accurate information system to retrieve, process, and report results in a timely manner; proper documentation of treatment with respect to previous radiographs or allergies; proper patient preparation for imaging examinations; proper imaging techniques (as measured by repeat/reject rates); proper interpretation, dictation, and verification of reports; and proper preventive maintenance of equipment. A radiology facility cannot improve its services with outdated policies, procedures, or technology or with a structure that does not allow for staff involvement in decision making. Investment in, and proper training of, staff members will broaden their assessment, communication, and clinical knowledge skills.

Point 2: Adopt the new philosophy.

The facility must be diligent and continue to improve the quality of radiology, provide a healthy environment in which to work, and be proud of the services given to the radiology patient. Radiology facilities need to have passionate medical direction, strong leadership, timely report turnaround times, modern technology, and highly trained technologists. With these attributes a facility can improve quality and efficiency and reduce costs.

Point 3: Cease dependence on mass inspection.

Inspecting the productivity of technologists based only on the number of radiologic procedures and images performed is counterproductive; the quality of the outcomes must be measured as well. The question to ask is, "Is there a quality outcome from the imaging exam?"

Point 4: End the practice of awarding business on price tag alone.

Buying higher quality items saves money and time in the long run. Further, businesses will tend to develop better quality items if such items are in demand. Using just-in-time delivery systems saves money and storage space, and it often resolves inventory or scheduling problems.

Point 5: Improve constantly and forever the system of production and service.

Every staff member in the radiology facility must work under the philosophy of continuous quality improvement (CQI). Fixing a problem halfway or not understanding the underlying root cause of a problem often creates bigger problems. CQI is a cycle of improvement; once a problem is fixed, the new process must be consistently monitored and analyzed.

Point 6: Institute training.

As healthcare and technology change, radiologists, technologists, and other clinical and support personnel within a radiology facility must be kept current on new treatments and practices. When facilities give or provide personnel the latest training, knowledge, and technology available, costs are reduced and the quality of clinical outcomes is increased.

Point 7: Institute leadership.

Leaders in heathcare manage staff and processes. Once managers learn QI skills, they can teach and lead by example. It is the radiology manager's role to provide staff members with adequate tools and time to give quality care to their patients.

Point 8: Drive out fear.

Staff members may not share concerns or point out problems to the radiology manager if they fear backlash from an attending physician, radiologist, or other healthcare provider. This situation can cause a lack of communication and lead to serious quality-of-care issues. Successful QI programs eliminate the fear associated with problem identification and encourage staff members to suggest ways to improve any and all aspects of their work environment.

Point 9: Break down barriers between departments and staff areas.

Interdepartmental communication is a must in quality care, because processes often involve more than one department. For example, hospital patients are routinely transported from nursing units to radiology, and communication problems could cause safety issues. The Joint Commission listed "hand off" communications as a National Patient Safety Goal for 2006 and similar goals should be expected in the future.

Point 10: Eliminate slogans, exhortations, and targets for the workforce.

Slogans developed by management without staff input are often not accepted by the staff members who are asked to use them. A QI program will help technologists and support staff develop their own goals, which will have more meaning for them.

Point 11: Eliminate quotas and other work standards.

Quotas may create an environment of inefficiency and reduced patient care. Under the pressure of meeting quotas, technologists may not have the time to listen to a patient or properly position a patient, resulting in an examination that is of poor diagnostic quality or that needs repeating. The focus should be on providing the best quality of care, not meeting a quota for examinations in a defined time period.

Point 12: Remove barriers to pride in workmanship.

When a quality program is successful in a radiology facility, the radiologists, technologists, and support staff are properly trained and have good avenues of communication. Staff members are normally motivated to do their job well, but they cannot do so if their training, technology, or work environment inhibits them. A QI program will identify these barriers and help eliminate them.

Point 13: Institute a vigorous program of education and retraining.

Radiology managers should be involved in the education and retraining of staff. A QI program budget should include adequate resources to train and retrain staff in QI techniques, methods, and job functions. Orientation programs should teach the basic policies and procedures and give an overview of the QI techniques.

Point 14: Take action to accomplish the transformation.

Radiology managers should recognize and admit to their own lack of quality in past performances and be able to adjust their style of management to improve the overall function of the facility. Adapting Deming's 14 points to processes and procedures within the facility will result in a workable QI program

Source: Cofer JI, Greeley HP, Wrinn MM. *Quality Improvement Techniques for Radiology: A Handbook.* Marblehead, MA: Opus IV Communications; 1993:17-23.

the world because it offered the latest technology, performed the greatest number of procedures by the greatest number of specialists, and had the fastest availability that money could buy.[4] As the postwar population began to age, more required heathcare and the cost of healthcare became an issue. The payors (industry and government) became concerned about the rise of healthcare costs in relation to the cost of living. To control this disparity, the value, quality, and cost equation was altered, thereby increasing value by lowering costs. Investigations of the healthcare system showed high utilization and many other causes for the rise in healthcare costs. These causes included new technology, an aging population, a legal environment leading to defensive medicine, administrative costs, and variations in efficiencies and quality of care.

Managed care emerged as a means to help control cost. Utilization review, quality assurance, and case management used by health maintenance organizations helped to relieve, but could not eliminate, the rising costs. Healthcare providers must now demonstrate the highest quality of care to knowledgeable patients with unlimited access to information about their care and treatment. With all these factors facing providers, quality has become important.

Today's performance improvement initiative is patient centered and performance focused as a functional orientation of healthcare organizations. Quality that does not include the customer usually does not produce a payoff in improved care, patient satisfaction, or market share. Healthcare today is driven by knowledgeable patients who insist on the best quality of care delivered efficiently and at the lowest cost possible.

Performance Measures and Indicators

A performance measure and indicator is a tool that provides an indication of a radiology facility's performance in relation to a specified process or outcome. For example, the technologists' repeat rates are measured and compared with national standards each month. A favorable outcome indicates that the technologists are performing within the national standards and patients are not being exposed to unnecessary radiation because of repeated exams. Performance measures relate to specific dimensions of care, treatment, and services provided, such as efficacy, appropriateness, availability, timeliness, effectiveness, continuity, safety, efficiency, and respect and caring. The Sidebar below describes these nine dimensions of performance and how they relate to radiology.[5]

SIDEBAR: The Nine Dimensions of Performance

Efficacy: The degree to which patient care has actually achieved the desired outcome.

A patient comes in for a diagnostic biopsy under imaging guidance. The specimen report is satisfactory for interpretation from the pathologist and is communicated to the referring physician.

Appropriateness: The degree to which the care and services provided are relevant to an individual's clinical needs.

All radiology examinations have medical necessity review before being completed.

Availability: The degree to which appropriate care and services can be accessed by the individual.

Imaging procedures will be available to the patient when necessary for quality of care.

Timeliness: The degree to which care is provided to a patient at the most beneficial or necessary time.

Imaging procedures will be performed when ordered by the referring physician and be reported immediately, if necessary.

Effectiveness: The degree to which care is provided correctly, given the current state of knowledge, to achieve the desired outcomes for the patient.

The appropriate modality will be used to accurately diagnose and treat the patient.

Continuity: The degree to which patient care is coordinated among practitioners, organizations, and time.

The radiology facility will be available to schedule and receive patients as necessary for quality care.

Safety: The degree to which the risk of an intervention and risk in the care environment are reduced for patients and others.

The radiology facility will guard against unnecessary radiation exposure to patients and their families, as well as to staff members.

Efficiency: The relationship between the outcomes and the resources used to deliver care (cost versus benefit).

The radiology facility will ensure the quality of care is efficiently performed with the appropriate equipment, staff, and supplies.

Respect and Caring: The degree to which individuals providing care and services do so with sensitivity to the patient's needs, expectations, and individual differences and the degree to which the patient is involved in his or her own care decisions.

The imaging technologist will instruct and educate patients about procedures being performed.

Source: Graham J, ed. *Collecting Data Efficiently.* Oakbrook Terrace, IL: The Joint Commission; 2004:57.

Monitoring Processes

A process is a sequence of tasks directed at accomplishing one particular outcome. In imaging, many processes occur to produce a diagnostic image, with the outcome being a quality diagnostic reading by the radiologist.

Processes have specific steps that everyone involved should understand, including where those steps fit into the larger picture. United in a common understanding, staff members can define starting and ending points of a process and figure out what has to happen in between to produce the necessary outcome. Everyone can focus on errors, waste, and other problems and determine what data will help them improve the effectiveness of this collection of tasks.

The processes are monitored through quality control measurements. With the collection of consistent data, analysis can determine if the desired outcome has been achieved. QI is realized when the entire process is improved to provide the best possible outcome for the patient.

Radiology administrators should evaluate the systems within their own facilities. The following are good questions to ask:

- What do we want to get out of this process?
- What do we have coming in?
- What must we do to get from one point to the other?
- What do we do that is necessary to reach our goals?
- Which steps are unnecessary?
- Where do we run into problems?

People who view work as processes understand how the quality of what comes out is largely determined by the quality of what goes in. How well technologists can do their jobs depends on the quality of the equipment and training they receive. And everyone depends on the policies, methods, tools, and equipment provided by managers. Quality is an organization-wide commitment starting with leadership development carried out by the facility as a whole.

If a series of related tasks can be called a *process*, a group of related processes can then be seen as a *system*. In radiology, related processes are procedures or examinations. A group of modality-specific procedures is a department.

Prioritizing Processes—Although healthcare workers may believe that everything they do is important, only those activities that are appropriate and essential to achieving the desired outcomes are of greatest importance. Choosing to measure only the important processes streamlines the appraisal process and makes the best use of resources.[1] Because healthcare facilities are complex systems, key function areas—which include direct patient care, management, and support processes and functions—have been identified by accrediting bodies for review.

Types of Processes—Not all processes are equal; some are critical and given immediate attention by a QI team. To assist an organization in developing a performance management system, predetermined criteria against which to measure and prioritize each process can be identified as high risk, high volume, problem prone, and high cost.

High risk describes an important process, procedure, or activity that exposes a patient to a greater chance of undesirable outcomes if not carried out effectively or appropriately. A process is high risk if its performance or omission could result in trauma, death, litigation, or loss of accreditation or license. In a radiology facility, interventional procedures are considered high risk, especially if they involve conscious sedation. High risk governance processes include failure to ensure licensure and credentialing of technical staff and lack of properly maintained disposable containers for used sharps.

High volume describes a process, procedure, or activity that is performed frequently or that affects large numbers of patients. Chest radiography is an example of a high volume procedure.

Problem prone describes a process, procedure, or activity that may have a high risk of problems. For example, a procedure may be a problem for patients who do not receive the correct preparation instructions. For the radiology manager, a problem prone process might be staff members' responding to a fire and safety code correctly. Anywhere a problem prone process, procedure, or activity is in place, consistent monitoring is essential.

High cost describes a process, procedure, or activity that may include items not covered by insurance or an invasive procedure requiring expensive supplies. Because healthcare costs are rising each year and the burden is being placed on the patient, facilities must pay attention to fiscal responsibility.

Plan Do Check Act (PDCA) Method

Walter Shewhart developed the Plan Do Check Act (PDCA) method of performance measurement in the 1920s. Shewhart was a pioneer in statistical quality control. Deming popularized this method in Japanese manufacturing plants during the rebuilding of Japan after World War II.

The PDCA method is a QI tool that focuses on one problem and then tests a solution. This method directs a team through the complete QI process, from identifying the main problem to implementing a solution and monitoring its continuous progress. The PDCA method is used to generate ideas and data to enhance planning, implementing, and monitoring. These steps define a problem, develop solutions, and clarify ideas on how to improve the problem (Box 3.1).

During the *Plan* phase of the cycle, the identified problem is analyzed. Brainstorming sessions should be used to narrow down the reasons or causes for the problem. At this time a process goal and proposed system solutions should be identified. Data from the existing system should be collected and analyzed (if not already done).

The *Do* phase of the cycle is the phase for implementing the solution or solutions identified in the Plan phase. Staff should be educated; costs and resources necessary

Box 3.1 Plan, Do, Check, Act (PDCA) Method

<table>
<tr><td>

ACT — Step 4

- Implement revised policies.
- Train staff on new procedures.
- Coordinate new standards with team leaders.
- Monitor new implementation.
- Revise and improve as needed.

</td><td>

PLAN — Step 1

- Analyze the identified issue.
- Develop an outcome goal.
- Identify data needed to monitor and analyze the issue.
- Consider quality improvement tools for data collection and organization.
- Finalize the action plan.

</td></tr>
<tr><td>

CHECK — Step 3

- Monitor and collect data.
- Meet with the team frequently to discuss the new plan.
- Use QI tools for collection and organization.
- Compare new data against old data for improvements in the process.
- Ask the team, "Is this working?"

</td><td>

DO — Step 2

- Think the plan through.
- Install any new equipment necessary to implement the plan.
- Instruct involved staff members.
- Conduct a test run and retrain, if needed.
- Document new procedures.

</td></tr>
</table>

Source: Adapted from Plan, Do, Check, Act Method, developed by Walter Shewhart focusing on one problem and then tests a solution. In: Cofer JI, Greeley HP, Wrinn MM. *Quality Improvement Techniques for Radiology: A Handbook.* Marblehead, MA: Opus IV Communications; 1993:81-84.

to implement the plan should be identified. Finally, the solution should be tested with a trial run before the existing system is changed.

During the *Check* phase, the newly implemented plan is monitored for improvements to the system. Meetings with staff are used to discuss changes, either negative or positive. QI tools such as Pareto charts, control charts, run charts, and surveys are used to collect data on the new system. After a thorough analysis, the success or failure of the solution is determined.

During the *Act* phase, the plan is incorporated into the facility's policy or standards. The staff is informed and educated, and the new standards are distributed to all key individuals. Most important is a continuing watch for new problems to solve or ways to improve. After this phase, the Plan phase resumes and the cycle begins again.[3]

PROCESS Method

The PROCESS method of QI involves *planning* a purpose, team and project scope; *researching* the current situation; *organizing* data and doing a gap analysis; *creating* and trying improvement; *evaluating* trial results; *standardizing* the process; and *starting* over. Box 3.2 below outlines the activities in the each phase.

Measurement Tools

Process and Outcomes Functions

Problems are identified using Pareto charts, fishbone diagrams, histograms, and run charts. Data collection functions use check sheets. Intervention design functions use flowcharts. Process control uses control charts. Results are reported by way of

---

Box 3.2 Seven Steps to the PROCESS Model

The PROCESS Model

Specify the plan requirements and objectives.
    Identify who, what, when, and how.
Analyze current processes.
    Identify the needs of the customers.
    Collect historical information.
Perform a root cause analysis.
    Display data is related graph form.
Identify improvement processes.
    Identify steps in the improved procedure.
    Develop a policy for the new process.
    Implement the new process.
Analyze the process.
    Collect data on implemented processes.
    Measure data using QI tools (graphs and charts).
Assess the process against proven standards.
    Document the process.
    Educate and reeducate as needed.
Begin the process again.
    Continually measure and identify areas for improvement.

Source: Adapted from Graham J. *Cost-effective Performance Improvement in Hospitals.* Oakbrook Terrace, IL: The Joint Commission; 2004:96.

---

instrument panels and report cards. These tools have come to define the classic approach to QI, and they are used to ensure that each step in a QI process provides valid conclusions.

Problem identification tools define the source of variation in a process, allowing planning to decrease inappropriate variation and improve quality. The various charts and diagrams are used to validate the problems identified.

Pareto Chart

In QI, a Pareto chart provides facts needed for setting priorities. It organizes and displays information to show the relative importance of various problems or causes of problems (Figure 3.1). It is essentially a special form of vertical bar chart that puts items in order (from the highest to the lowest) relative to some measurable effect of interest (for example, frequency, cost, or time). The chart is based on the Pareto principle, which states that when several factors affect a situation, a few factors will account for most of the impact. The Pareto principle describes a phenomenon in which 80% of variation observed in everyday processes can be explained by a mere 20% of the causes of that variation.

Placing the items in descending order of frequency makes it easy to discern the problems that are of greatest importance or the causes that appear to account for

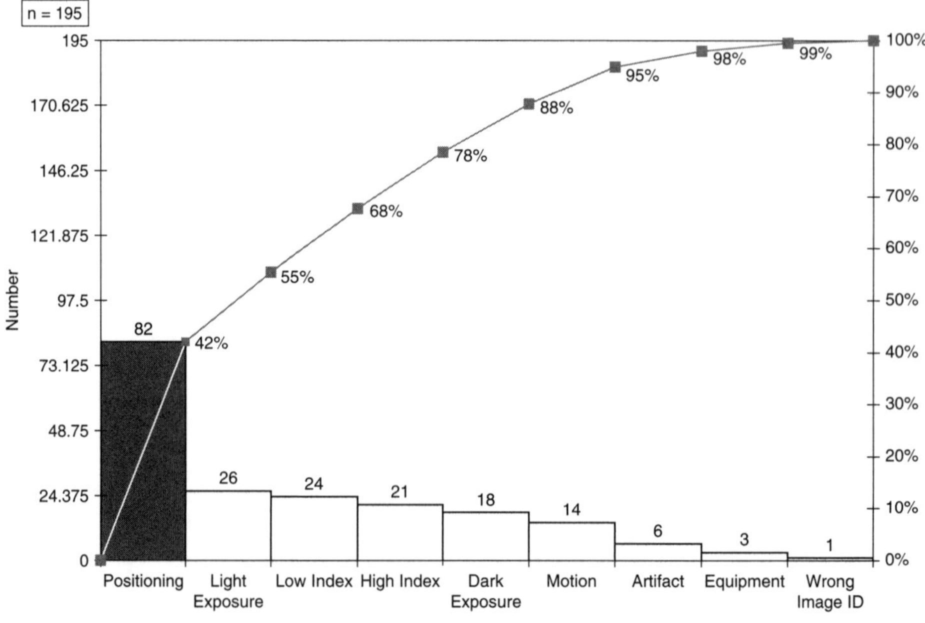

Figure 3.1 A Pareto chart.

most of the variation. Thus, a Pareto chart helps teams to focus their efforts where they can have the greatest potential impact.

Pareto charts help teams focus on the small number of really important problems or causes of problems. Pareto charts are useful in establishing priorities by identifying the most critical problems to be tackled or causes to be addressed. Comparing Pareto charts of a given situation over time can also determine whether an implemented solution reduced the relative frequency or cost of that problem or cause.[6]

In short, Pareto charts are used for the following:

- Focusing on areas of priority.
- Prioritizing factors and putting them in graphic form simply and quickly.

Other Charts

The *fishbone diagram* is another cause-and-effect method whereby the step-by-step process is followed from beginning to end in order to look at each stage of production. This diagram is often referred to as a pictorial display of a list (Figure 3.2). It is useful in a team meeting or brainstorming session. Root causes are discovered more effectively in a large group of staff members who are close to the process in question.

A *histogram chart* is a bar graph that displays data over time. The chart uses raw data, putting the class intervals on the horizontal (x) axis and frequency on the vertical (y) axis. The histogram is used to analyze a process with variable results in its data. The information received will determine if process adjustments create a positive or negative impact. It is best to implement this tool when at least 40 data items can be used.

An example is the number of chest radiographs in a week and the number of minutes it took to complete the procedure, interpret the radiograph, dictate, and deliver the report to the referring physician. The chart may be bell shaped, be skewed, or have twin

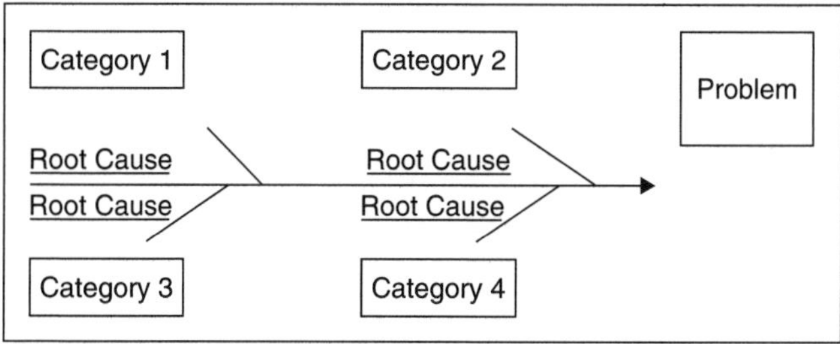

**Figure 3.2 A cause-and-effect (fishbone) diagram used
to identify problems in a process.**

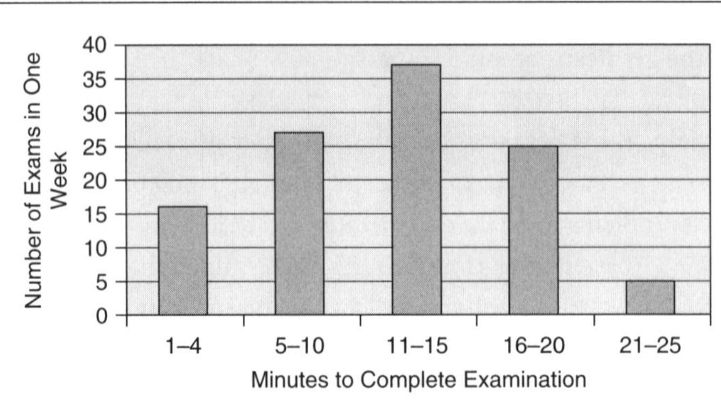

Number of Exams in 1 Week

Class Intervals	Number of Exams in 1 Week							
Minutes to complete examination	Mon	Tue	Wed	Thu	Fri	Sat	Sun	Total
1-4	2	4	5	2	1		2	16
5-10	3	4	5	5	6	3	1	27
11-15	4	8	6	4	7	3	5	37
16-20	3	2	5	6	3	3	3	25
21-25			3		1		1	5

Figure 3.3 A histogram displaying data over time.

peaks (be bimodal). When all the data are consistently in the middle of the chart, spread evenly, the distribution is considered to be a bell shape, with normal expectations of a process. Positively and negatively skewed histograms reflect a process that has variables that cannot be changed. If it is skewed to the right, it is negatively skewed; if it is skewed to the left, it is positively skewed. Twin peaks indicate that either something is wrong with the data or the data come from two different sources. Figure 3.3 is an example of a bell-shaped histogram with normal expectations for the minutes it took to complete a chest radiograph for a period of 1 week.

Run charts show data plotted over time. This simple method is used for analyzing trends, shifts, or changes in a process.

Interventional design makes use of the fact that variation in a process exists because the process does not operate the same way every time. To get a handle on how the system ideally operates or should operate, standardization of the process must occur.

Flowcharts can be extremely valuable for radiology managers in understanding and optimizing processes. Often, the very act of producing a flowchart reveals problems in process flow that respond to simple intervention. In more complex

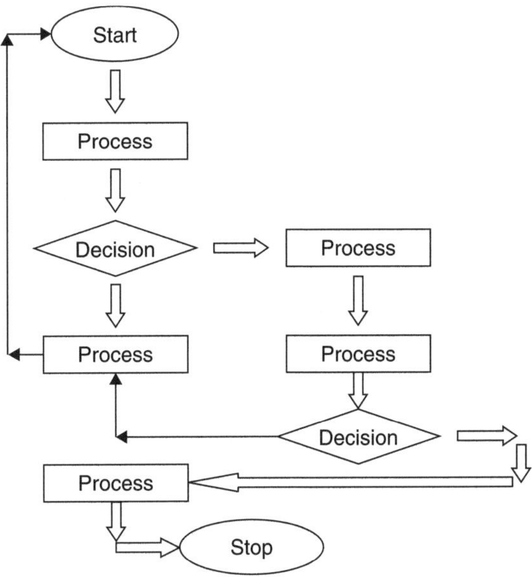

Figure 3.4 A flowchart.

processes, flowcharting may present the only means of understanding the true structure of a system (Figure 3.4).

Many consider process control to be the most critical measure of QI. Through the use of statistical process *control charts*, data can be expressed in terms of means and up to three standard deviations above and below those means, over which data collection points are plotted. Based on these data points, variations in the process that are outside expected limits can be identified and targeted for intervention. Control charts are most useful for ongoing processes in which variation is a source of cost and diminished productivity; these statistical models allow rapid analysis and intervention for active processes (Figure 3.5). In radiology, control charts are useful for analyzing performance and outcome measures in diagnostic and therapeutic systems of care for specific disorders or preventive care. Using control charts, radiology managers can usually identify sources of variation that determine approaches for

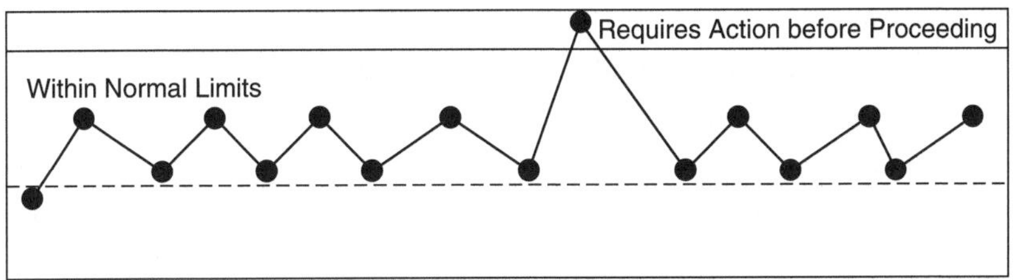

Figure 3.5 A control chart This chart shows data within normal limits and one data point outside the normal limits requiring action before the process can proceed.

improvement. Control charts are typically used in darkroom quality control plans to monitor imaging processors. Mammography programs must chart the processor quality control before performing mammography each day.

Instrument Panels

Pareto charts and control charts display frequencies of events and outcomes. In a QI project, the radiology manager or the process improvement team often chooses key variables and groups these data displays in an array of multiple figures or tables that capture the procedures and processes. These instrument panels (1) illustrate real-time monitoring as action is taking place, (2) present information that is dynamic and occurring in real time that may target future goals, and (3) empower the individuals improving the process through informed decision making. A healthcare instrument panel is a display of data, perhaps histograms and control charts, that would advise and monitor a QI team's efforts to maintain and improve the quality of processed images. In summary, instrument panels convey a careful and thoughtful approach to the display of data that is helpful in stimulating action toward a goal.

Report Cards

During QI work, a radiology manager may be asked to present information, such as outcomes data, in the form of charts or instrument panels to upper management, corporate boards or leadership, accrediting bodies such as The Joint Commission or the MQSA, or regulatory agencies at the state or federal levels. These information displays usually report results that demonstrate accountability for care. They usually display past successes or a lack thereof. This display of data (1) is somewhat static; (2) usually reflects past summaries of information; (3) shows results that may be open to judgment and may produce apprehension, rejection, or sometimes joy; and (4) centers around conclusions about outcomes on or around average expectations. An example of a report card in radiology would be the MQSA medical outcomes audit completed annually for accredited mammography facilities.

Methods: Root Cause Analysis

Good intentions, teamwork, data acquisition and analysis, and changes tested in improvement cycles are all essential to improving healthcare. All too often, the focus on improvement results in personal "shame or blame." When, in actuality, failures may likely be due to process or system deficiencies that lead to inefficiencies, error, or poor results. Flowcharts can help the manager visualize the process that exists. However, in healthcare, processes and systems are extremely complex and even at times chaotic. These complex process interactions in systems are best evaluated using the method known as *root cause analysis (RCA)*.

RCA can help individuals learn as much as possible from adverse events or poor outcomes of processes in systems. It is not enough to just learn about what happened when expectations failed to be met. It is more important to know why something happened and to learn how to prevent a recurrence. A root cause is the most basic reason a situation did not turn out ideally. Most often, a root cause is a known or unknown system vulnerability (human weakness is almost never a root cause). The evaluation of root causes involves a rigorous, thoughtful team approach to flow diagramming and construction of cause-and-effect diagrams after consideration of (1) failures in human factors of communication, training, and fatigue or scheduling; (2) environmental or equipment failures; (3) factors relating to rules, policies, or procedures; and (4) barriers. One enters into each of these areas of consideration asking the question "why" multiple times, thus delving deeply into each process or system interaction beyond simple explanations.

Evolving Practices and Initiatives

The historic context of the manufacturing and service sectors of the economy have influenced the tools and methods being applied to healthcare system quality management. Within the business community, a multitude of process improvement champions seem to be vying for attention and leading others toward a "best" method. Each champion advocates the adoption of his or her favored improvement methodology. Three current methodologies are six sigma, lean thinking, and the theory of constraints (TOC). As is usually the case, no one method is best for all situations. These programs, their application, and their implementation are worthy of brief discussion. In addition, the business improvement programs of the Baldrige Awards and the principles involved in the management of high-reliability organizations (nuclear power plants, aviation, and aerospace) are entering the environment of healthcare as coalitions of businesses, payors, providers, and regulators come together. A brief summary of these programs and principles follows.

Six Sigma

Six sigma refers to the statistical likelihood that there will be only 3.4 failures or defects in a million opportunities. This quality management method was first implemented at Motorola. In addition, it has been popularized by tremendous successes in management at General Electric. Some experts believe the method should be equally as successful in healthcare. Reduction of variation in the areas of medication administration, surgical procedures, assignment of caregivers, emergency treatment triage, patient falls, and disease management are just a few applications where the DMAIC guidelines (define, measure, analyze, improve, and control) of six sigma resemble and complement PDSA cycles of improvement. The focus of six sigma centers on reducing, and ideally removing, failure and defects within work processes.

Lean Thinking

Lean thinking is sometimes called *lean manufacturing* and was popularized in manufacturing by the Toyota production system. This method focuses on the removal of waste in work environments. *Waste* is defined as anything not necessary to produce the product or service. The common measure is *touch time*—the amount of time the product is actually being worked on or touched by the worker. Frequently, the focus of lean thinking is manifested in an emphasis on flow through a process. Five essential steps in the method are: (1) identify features that create value, (2) identify the sequence of activities called the *value stream*, (3) make the activities flow, (4) let the customer pull the product or service through the system, and (5) perfect the process. Recent collaboration between General Motors and its employees' healthcare providers has reduced costs and improved outcomes—truly a win-win for the purchaser, users, and providers of healthcare.

Theory of Constraints

TOC is the approach to continuous improvement based on a five-step procedure. These five steps are as follows: (1) identify the constraint (processes that may affect work flow), (2) exploit the constraint (increase the efficiency of the constraint process), (3) subordinate all other processes to the constraint process (put other process in place of the constraint), (4) elevate the constraint (monitor and collect data), and (5) repeat the process.

TOC looks at processes from a system point of view. All leaders and employees must understand the goal of the facility and have a commitment to quality that is based on understanding interrelationships and interdependencies. When using TOC as a way of implementing problem solving about a process, the continuous improvement programs are most effective and the solutions longer lasting.[7]

Baldrige Awards

The Malcolm Baldrige National Quality Award was created by Public Law 100-107 and signed into law on August 20, 1987. The award is named for Malcolm Baldrige, former secretary of commerce. Baldrige's managerial excellence contributed to long-term improvement in the efficiency and effectiveness of government. The award not only recognizes quality but also establishes a framework within which quality initiatives take place. Most organizations that apply for the award believe that even greater gains accrue through evaluating their systems than may result from being awarded one of the coveted awards. The Baldrige performance excellence criteria allow organizations to improve overall performance in seven categories: leadership, strategic planning, customer and market focus, information analysis, human resource focus, process management, and business results.

The Baldrige HealthCare Criteria are built on the following set of interrelated core values and concepts: visionary leadership, patient-focused excellence, organization and personal learning, valuing staff and partners, agility, focusing on the future, managing for innovation, management by fact, social responsibility and community health, focusing on results, and creating a value and systems perspective. The Baldrige HealthCare Criteria for Performance Excellence can be found online at http://www.quality.nist.gov/HealthCare_Criteria.htm.

High-Reliability Organizations—"Management of the Unexpected"

Lessons learned from other complex and error-prone environments can, and must, be applied to the management of healthcare systems. The aerospace, aviation, and nuclear energy industries—known as *high-reliability organizations (HROs)*—must consistently produce safe, reproducible, error-free services and products. The National Patient Safety Center has been charged with teaching applications of these principles and actions to reduce human and system error in healthcare organizations. Weick and Sutcliffe have described the five hallmarks of HROs: (1) a preoccupation with failure, (2) reluctance to simplify interpretations, (3) sensitivity to operations, (4) commitment to resilience, and (5) deference to expertise.[8] Tools for assessing an organization's preparation and implementation of "mindful management" are essential for the management of quality and error prevention in medical care systems.[4]

Data Collection

Data collection is an important activity in QI. In radiology, data collection can involve items as specific as control charts and as complex as interdepartmental customer satisfaction. Data are the foundation of a performance measurement program. Shewhart stated, "Knowledge begins with data and ends with other data."[5] He emphasized the importance of data in building knowledge.

During quality control, the radiology facility collects data on processor performance, lead apron integrity, contrast warmer temperatures, crash cart daily checks, and more. Measurement of equipment performance is important to QI. Quality control is the process by which actual performance is measured.

Facilities need to identify processes that are inefficient and problem prone. Teams should form to track the performance of a process, discuss trends and patterns to improve the problem prone areas within a process, and then systematically fix the inefficient components of the process until the process is working smoothly.

Data are the documentation of observations and customer feedback, either verbal or written, over a designated period. Data are categorized into two types, objective and subjective. Objective data are data on charts and check sheets completed by staff members when they perform a procedure or complete a task. Subjective data are information received from patient surveys and feedback from suggestion boxes, such as perceived satisfaction or feelings. It is important to remember that the process and outcome must be the driving forces behind data collection. Data collection must be linked to an outcome, and a process should be improved or declared satisfactory if the data collection process is to be efficient and useful.

Planning for Data Collection

Any time a radiology administrator collects data, a team should be in place to review the process in question. The data collection should reveal opportunities, confirm variations in process performance, track data and identify trends, predict future performance, and confirm the success of any changes made to the process. The team of staff members who are touched by the process under analysis should be given the following questions to answer before data collection begins:

- What are the goals for collecting these data?
- Who should collect the data?
- In which domain should the data be collected?
- For what purpose should the data be collected?
- What are the data sources?
- How much data should be collected?
- What tools will be used?
- What bias exists?

Because data collection is such an important task in performance improvement, the following goals should be established for the team:

- Ensure the accuracy of information on which to base future decisions. A poor decision based on inaccurate data can be extremely costly to the organization.
- Avoid punitive measures associated with the result of collected data. Employees will cooperate with collecting and organizing data when they feel secure and unafraid of retaliation and negative consequences.
- Pinpoint the exact area of the facility that contains the performance opportunities.

- Establish the degree to which improvement occurred after the implementation of an improvement action plan.
- Collect data at regular intervals on all critical processes to demonstrate sustained improvement.
- Collect both subjective and objective data.[1]

Purpose of Data Collection

Data are collected for four major reasons. First, data that shows a positive outcome and high level of customer satisfaction demonstrate that the organization-wide performance management system is functioning well. Second, data should provide a basis for change or improvement in the service provided. Accurate data will lay the foundation for necessary change and continual improvement. Third, the data should provide a rationale for increased or decreased resources within the facility. Fourth, the data should provide a basis for development of reliable performance improvement targets for evaluation to be used in tracking and analyzing trends.

Sources of Data

Data sources are categorized into three types: the consumer, the healthcare provider, and the management of the provider. All three contain important data elements, and each must be considered when planning and implementing a QI process. Examples of the three types of sources in a radiology facility are the patients and their families; the staff members; and the management sources that include department leadership, supervisors, top management, and the board of directors.

Amount of Data

It would be unrealistic to collect data on all processes and procedures in a radiology facility. Target parameters have been established for various data collection reasons. The Katz-Green guidelines for data collection states the following:

- *Routine review of data.* The sample size should be 5% or 30 (whichever is greater).
- *Query review of data.* The sample size should be 10% or 60 (whichever is greater).
- *Intensive review of data.* The sample size should be 15% or 90 (whichever is greater).
- *Sentinel event.* The sample size should be 100% (every event).[1]

Evaluation of Data

Data that have been collected are considered raw data until they are aggregated and analyzed. Many of the measurement tools in this chapter are used to collect the data, keep it organized, and give a pictorial image of the processes being investigated. Once a variation is discovered, the source type must be identified. If a service variable is the cause, a customer/family action plan is needed to address scheduling, patient education, or preparation. If service variables are not the cause, staff or management variables are looked at. It may also be possible that all three types of variables contribute to the variation found in the data collection process. Once the analysis has been completed, the planning and trial phase of the revised processes can take place.

Resources/Accrediting Bodies and Regulations

Radiology administrators should understand resources for quality and know where to find them. Many organizations provide information on healthcare quality for professionals and consumers. Publications and information on the Internet are available and can provide a wealth of information to structure a quality program in the facility.

The following organizations are working to improve the quality of care given to all patients and families in US hospitals:

- AARP
- AFL/CIO
- Agency for Healthcare Research and Quality
- American Hospital Association
- American Medical Association
- Association of American Medical Colleges
- Centers for Medicare and Medicaid Services
- Consumer-Purchaser Disclosure Project
- Federation of American Hospitals
- The Joint Commission
- National Association of Children's Hospitals and Related Institutions
- National Quality Forum
- US Chamber of Commerce

In addition to this list, there are many organizations that are interested in hospital quality and are working with the above groups to improve the quality of care in the US. Some of these groups are:

- State survey agencies in every state
- Quality improvement organizations (QIO) in every state
- American Osteopathic Association
- US Department of Veterans Affairs

Radiology organizations, such as the American College of Radiology (ACR) and the Mammography Quality Standards Act (MQSA), provide criteria specific to radiology facilities. The MQSA regulations provide quality standards for facilities to ensure safe, reliable, and accurate mammography. The regulations set under the MQSA rules do not apply to facilities of the US Department of Veterans Affairs.

The ACR consists of radiologists, radiation oncologists, medical physicists, interventional radiologists, and nuclear medicine physicians. The ACR quality resources available to radiology administrators provide information on accreditation processes and ACR appropriateness criteria, which are evidence-based guidelines to assist referring physicians and other healthcare providers in making appropriate imaging or treatment decisions. Providers use these guidelines to enhance quality of care and contribute to the most effective use of radiology.[9]

Modalities available for accreditation through the ACR are mammography, radiation oncology, MRI, nuclear medicine and PET, breast ultrasonography, stereotactic breast biopsy, CT, and ultrasonography. These programs are voluntary and confer many benefits on facilities seeking the ACR accreditation. These benefits include a demonstration of peer review; qualified personnel and equipment; assessment of image quality; marketing tools; and help in meeting specific criteria of the American Cancer Society, government agencies, and third-party payors. Contact information for these resources appears in Table 3.1.

Staff Empowerment and QI

Staff commitment to QI starts at the top. The CEO and governing boards must be committed and open to empowering staff in team processes and resources to resolve problems. In turn, staff members will work in an environment of continuous improvement. Technologists and support staff often know their job duties better than anyone in the facility. This hands-on experience provides an awareness of performance improvement opportunities unknown by many managers. Technologists who have worked at other facilities may have ideas from them that can improve quality.

Once empowered, employees begin to take pride and ownership in their work. Doing so may lead to improvement in job performance, which then may increase overall organizational quality. All employees should be enlisted to collect data regarding processes in their areas, such as pain assessment and effective management, procedure documentation, or compliance with hand washing.

Table 3.1 Organization List

Resource	Purpose	Web Address
American Cancer Society	Cancer statistics and information	www.cancer.org
American Hospital Association	Hospital information	www.aha.org
American Medical Association	Physician information	www.ama-assn.org
Association of American Medical Colleges	Hospital information	www.aamc.org
Centers for Medicare & Medicaid Services	Information about Medicare coverage	For Professionals: www.cms.hhs.gov For Consumers: www.medicare.gov
Federation of American Hospitals	Hospital information	www.fah.org
Food and Drug Administration	Regulations	www.fda.gov
The Joint Commission	Hospital performance reports	www.jointcommission.org
Mammography Quality Standards Act	Mammography standards	www.fda.gov/cdrh/mammography/index.html
National Association of Children's Hospitals and Related Institutions	Information about children's healthcare quality	www.childrenshospitals.net
National Guidelines Clearinghouse	Resource for evidence-based clinical practice guidelines	www.ngc.gov

Conclusion

The knowledge of QI is crucial for radiology managers to effectively promote efficient, high-quality, high-valued healthcare. Patients, referring physicians, and regulators are demanding, and will continue to demand, performance-based data that document an understanding, application, and implementation of QI principles with regard to the services that they need and expect.

The reason for a QI plan is to monitor processes and reduce the inevitable human error. Physicians and staff members must understand how to reduce the impact of human error in the process of delivering patient care safely. Quality tools and techniques should be used to measure and analyze performance and to implement improved processes. Errors, either human or system related, should be managed through culture changes, strategies, and improved process designs. To maintain a level of acceptable quality, the facility must commit to tracking progress against desired goals, identifying new opportunities, and comparing performance with internal and external benchmarks. Incidence reports, physician and patient surveys, regulatory surveys, and QI data are essential tools in data collection.

Identifying what to measure is critical. Each facility should answer the following questions when selecting performance measures:

- In a hospital, are the radiology department's services contributing to the organization's overall success through the achievement of strategic goals? How can the department's contribution be measured?
- What performance does the facility want to improve? What critical activities and outcomes should be measured?
- What are the vital requirements of the facility's customers? What is most important to patients and other internal customers? How can these customer expectations be measured?
- What is important to accreditation and regulatory agencies? What are the national or local topics of interest that affect patient care services, and how can these issues be measured?[10]

Once data have been collected, the radiology manager must measure the data and react to them in a constructive way. The goal should be realistic, promote high quality, create a safe environment, and steer away from impossible processes that discourage and stifle productivity.

Analyzing the results of measured data is a crucial component in the improvement process. The data should be timely, concise, and relevant to the service being provided. The results should provide information on how current performance compares with the intended outcomes of the specific improvement process activity. Factors that should be taken into consideration when analyzing data include the right measurements; organization-wide priorities; trend identification; and improvements that target cost saving, QI, safety, or all three.

Once the data have been collected, measured, and analyzed, the radiology manager must share the results with physicians, staff members, and other key managers. If results are not used, employees may not take management seriously; all the time and effort put into the quality process will be wasted. When leaders and staff in the facility take QI seriously, the results can be enormous.

The return on time invested in quality is using the data to improve processes and performance. Learn from the pioneers of quality, use the tools, and communicate the information to the staff and leaders who can make the process better. Having a culture of excellence starts with a healthy work environment where there is a mutual respect between management and staff working together toward the best patient care.

References

1. Katz JM, Green E. *Managing Quality: A Guide to System Wide Performance Management in Health Care.* 2nd ed. New York, NY: Mosby–Year Book; 1997.

2. Crosby P. The fun uncle of the quality revolution. Available at: http://www.skymark.com/resources/leaders/crosby.asp. Accessed February 26, 2006.

3. Cofer JI, Greeley HP, Wrinn MM. *Quality Improvement Techniques for Radiology: A Handbook.* Marblehead, MA: Opus IV Communications; 1993: 17–23.

4. Bennett S, Slavin L. Continuous quality improvement: what every health care manager needs to know. Available at: http://www.case.edu/med/epidbio/mphp439/CQI.htm. Accessed February 26, 2006.

5. Graham J, ed. *Collecting Data Efficiently.* Oakbrook Terrace, IL: The Joint Commission; 2004:57.

6. Quality Assurance Project. Pareto chart. Available at: http://www.qaproject.org/methods/resparetochart.html. Accessed March 19, 2006.

7. Theory of constraints. Available at: http://www.optimums.com/inqualtocpop.htm. Accessed March 10, 2007.

8. Weick K, Sutcliffe K. Managing the unexpected. San Francisco: Jossey-Bass. 2001.

9. ACR appropriateness criteria. Available at: http://www.acr.org/s_acr/sec.asp?CID=1845& DID=16050. Accessed October 13, 2006.

10. Spath, P. Process improvement. *Radiology Today,* 2006; 7:17. Available at: http://www.radiologytoday.net/archive/rt11606p17.shtml. Accessed February 26, 2006.

Chapter 4

Identifying Resources

Robert P. Brice

Creating a strategic plan and setting goals are fundamental to ensuring the growth and success of a facility or radiology department. Yet no plan can be carried out without expending resources, including financial, technological, and human resources. Thus, it is critical to identify the resources that will be available to meet goals and achieve the strategic plan.

Identifying Financial Resources

Few goals can be achieved without some level of financing. Whereas plans to purchase capital equipment will likely call for a financial commitment beyond the facility's balance sheet, the radiology administrator in a well-run facility will often find the financial resources to carry out other plans in cash reserves, profits, revenue growth, and budget savings. Among the ways to identify these resources are carrying out financial trend (historical) analysis, forecasting revenue and profits, and exploring alternative sources. (For a more detailed discussion of financial aspects of strategic planning, refer to *Financial Management in Radiology.*[1])

Examining the Past

A facility that has experienced a consistent growth in profits over the past 3 years can plan for the coming year with some confidence. Trend analysis and other assessments carried out to develop a strategic plan, as discussed in Chapter 1, may also be helpful in analyzing the facility's financial history. Radiology administrators can collect data for this analysis from various sources, including specialized radiology management software, the CFO and accounting/business office staff, and departmental patient check-in sheets. A key driver of radiology revenues is volume, usually tracked through procedures or Current Procedural Terminology (CPT) codes. Reviewing volume by CPT code on a year-to-date basis for the past 2 to 3 years can determine the facility's historical growth rate. Taking the average of 3 years' rates produces a projected volume growth rate for the coming year.

Most facilities experience seasonal rises and dips in volume. Calculating the seasonality index based on past volume can help in timing the implementation of new projects or goals that may depend on increased revenues. To develop a seasonality index, use these steps:

1. Collect volume data by month for the past 3 years.
2. Calculate the average volume for each month over the 3-year period.
3. Add the average volumes together and divide by 12 to get the average monthly volume.
4. Divide each month's average volume by the average monthly volume to get each month's seasonal index.

The higher the index number, the greater the volume (and, presumably, the revenues) for that month.

Any of several business ratios can provide insight into current-year financial health and the potential for revenues to be available to achieve goals. Some ratios are more valuable to freestanding, for-profit imaging centers than to nonprofit organizations or hospital-based departments. The following ratios are among the more useful:

- *Current ratio*—Calculated by dividing current assets by current liabilities, the current ratio reflects the facility's ability to meet its accounts payables for the near future. Although it is best that the ratio be 1 or higher, a higher-than-normal number may indicate an accounts receivable collection problem.
- *Total debt ratio*—Calculated simply by dividing the total amount of outstanding debt by total assets, the total debt ratio indicates the business's solvency. The lower the number, the lower the leverage. Less debt leaves more capital for growth, projects, and other goals; too much debt is a prescription for bankruptcy. The total debt ratio is an important factor in seeking financing for capital equipment purchases or other long-term debt.
- *Profit margin*—Calculated by dividing net income by revenue, the profit margin (also known as the *total margin*) reflects the rate at which the business has money left after all expenses to invest in capital equipment and other means to business growth.
- *Return on assets ratio*—Calculated by dividing net income by total assets, the return on assets ratio is a measure of how effectively the business is using its assets to generate profit.
- *Days in accounts receivable*—Calculated by multiplying the net patient receivables by 365, then dividing by the net patient revenue, the resulting days in accounts receivable is the average collection time. A high number may reflect poor collection policies or other problems in accounts receivable. It also means that cash will not be available in a timely fashion for use in carrying out the strategic plan.

An individual facility's ratios can be compared with industry standards. For purposes of identifying available financial resources for goals and projects, however, the radiology administrator will find trend analysis over time more useful. Comparing the current year's ratio to the ratios of the previous 2 or 3 years can reveal whether the facility is improving financially and whether funds are likely to be available.

Forecasting Revenue and Profit

Past performance, of course, is no guarantee of future performance. Any effort to identify financial resources to achieve goals must include forecasts of revenue and profit. Some of the ratios previously described—such as total debt ratio—when applied to the current year, provide clues to the level of funding that may be carried over into the next year. Application of the seasonality index to the average number of procedures expected for each month in the coming year will reveal periods most likely to generate excess revenue.

Much of the analysis performed to establish goals and determine needs (see Chapter 2) can be put to further use in assessing financial resources. Every projected change, at its most basic level, should be analyzed for its financial impact. For example, if a radiologist's contract expires and is not renewed, revenues will decline until a replacement is found, but so will salaries and expenses related to the physician's activities. A procedure that recently replaced an outmoded one may generate substantially more revenue if it is reimbursed at a higher rate, is performed substantially more often, or has much lower expenses related to carrying it than did the discontinued procedure. (See Box 4.1).

Box 4.1 A Pro Forma Forecasts Success

Being able to accurately forecast the financial results of a planned expansion, proposed new modality, or other major project is the key to obtaining financial support. A pro forma is a set of financial statements that presents the radiology administrator's best estimate of a project's potential impact in the coming years (usually 3 to 5 years). The pro forma can help "sell" the project to senior management, as well as potential funders. Putting it together can also be a valuable tool in the initial decision about whether to proceed with the project.

The following are the key elements in the pro forma document :

1. Income projections for 3 to 5 years, based on current ratios, local trends, and estimates of the project's impact on business growth.
2. The break-even point—the point at which the project's revenues will be equal to the expenses incurred.
3. A projected balance sheet indicating assets, liabilities, and net assets for the 3- to-5-year time horizon.
4. The return on investment—that is, the percentage found by dividing the net return of the project by the total investment used to fund it.

Development of pro forma projections (or forecast) allows for the exploration of various scenarios, using actual costs when available and estimating cost projections based on other resources. Estimates can often be provided by vendors and/or industry articles or surveys. By changing parameters such as volume or staffing costs, the manager is able to determine when equipment might pay for itself.

Calculating a staffing budget is another tool that identifies whether revenues will be available for goals. Staffing levels are generally based on the concept of a full-time equivalent, or FTE, which represents each 40 hours worked in a week (no matter by how many employees). The FTE/volume ratio is calculated by dividing the number of procedures performed (in a day, week, month, or year) by the number of FTEs used to carry them out. This ratio then can be used to forecast the number of FTEs needed in the future.

For example, if 4 FTEs produce 2000 MRI procedures a month, the FTE/volume ratio is 500. If the radiology administrator forecasts increasing MRI output by 50%, to 3000 per month, then 2 more FTEs will be needed. Applying the salary assigned to the relevant job codes, including cost-of-living and merit raises and benefits, to the additional FTEs will yield a forecast of the increase in salary needed. In contrast, if the staffing mix changes because new procedures require fewer FTEs, funds may become available for new projects.

Identifying Alternative Sources of Financing

In most instances, projects within a strategic plan and short-term goals can be funded from profits and increased revenues generated by the projects themselves. However, larger projects, such as building a satellite office or installing PACS, put demands on finances that must be met by resources outside the facility (see Box 4.2). At least three types of funding sources are available: grants, debt capital, and equity capital. Although different, they share a common characteristic—they require a solid explanation of the project, how the funds will be used, and what will be given in exchange for funds.

Grants and Philanthropy—Radiology departments within nonprofit hospitals or other healthcare facilities may find grant funding for projects ranging from community outreach on mammography screening to expanding services for underserved populations. Unlike many other funding sources, grants do not have to be repaid, and so for purposes of this discussion they include funds raised through capital campaigns and other philanthropic efforts. The facility's development or fundraising staff may be able to help identify potential grantors or donors, as might the following resources:

Box 4.2 Small Business Administration: A Potential Source for Loans

The US Small Business Administration (SBA) has a number of loan programs available to small businesses; for services such as healthcare, the SBA defines small businesses as those with yearly receipts not exceeding $5 million. The SBA also requires that the business be for profit, independently owned, and not dominant in its field.

The SBA does not directly loan money. Rather, it guarantees loans given by commercial lenders and nonprofit agencies that it licenses and certifies. Among the SBA programs are 7(a) loan guarantees and the Microloan Program.

7(a) loan guarantees are one of the SBA most widely used programs, allowing small businesses that would otherwise not qualify for bank financing to borrow funds for renovations, equipment, construction of commercial buildings, or purchase of land or buildings. Rates vary with the size of the loan and the repayment schedule, but they are generally set a few percentage points above the prime rate. The assets being funded provide collateral. Application is through an SBA-certified bank, which handles all the processing, communication with the SBA, and fund dispersal and collection.

The popular Microloan Program works through certified nonprofit intermediaries to loan between $100 and $25,000. Funds can be used for equipment or renovations to existing facilities. Generally, rates are set at 4 percentage points above prime rate, and the assets being purchased serve as collateral.

To find out more about these SBA loan programs and others, the radiology administrator can consult www.sba.gov or check in the local telephone directory under "US Government" for the nearest regional SBA office.

Grantmakers in Health

www.gih.org

National Rural Health Association

www.nrharural.org

Office of Rural Health Policy

ruralhealth.hrsa.gov/funding

Robert Wood Johnson Foundation

www.rwjf.org

Agency for Healthcare Research and Quality

www.ahrq.gov/fund

Directory of Biomedical and Health Care Grants. Phoenix, AZ: Oryx Press; published annually.

Granting organizations, which include foundations, government agencies, and corporations, often fund specific categories of projects, such as expanding health services to rural communities or to children. One key to successfully getting a project funded is to identify how the project fits within the grantor's area of interest. The stronger the link, the greater the likelihood a grant will be awarded.

Generally, a grant application asks for the following:

- A general description of the organization, its services, and its patient base.
- A description of the project to be funded, including its projected impact.
- The amount needed, along with a detailed budget.
- Plans for additional or future funding to ensure the project's viability.

Most granting organizations have online applications with full instructions and tips for successful application.

Debt Capital—Commonly referred to as *loans*, debt capital is funds that are borrowed for a specified time and must be repaid, usually with interest. Although the loan may be secured by the facility's assets, the lender does not gain ownership rights.

Banks offer various types of loans (see Box 4.3), but the four most common types follow:

- A short-term loan, usually in the form of a promissory note, is primarily used for a specific, short-term project, with the loan payable at the end of the project.
- An operating line of credit provides capital "as needed" to a prespecified limit, with no interest charged until funds are used.
- An intermediate-term loan usually runs for 3 to 5 years and is used to purchase equipment, expand facilities, or even purchase another business. The loan is secured by the business's assets.
- A long-term loan is used to purchase land or major buildings, with the loan secured by the asset.

Box 4.3 Locating Sources of Financial Support: Get Creative

Sources of financial support are not always obvious. A radiology administrator who thinks creatively may find funds for a wide array of projects. Among the alternatives are vendor financing, cooperative arrangements, and corporate sponsorships.

Vendor financing. The major manufacturers of healthcare and business equipment can provide funds to purchase their equipment, usually through a subsidiary. Among these sources are GE Capital Corporation (for GE Healthcare and other equipment; www.gecapital.com), Hewlett-Packard (for high-tech equipment; www.hp.com), and Oracle Credit Corporation (for computers and software; www.oracle.com).

Cooperative arrangements. Projects may be funded in cooperation with another business. For example, a series of lectures by the facility's staff might be presented at a local mall's community room, with the mall providing the room and advertising in local newspapers. A printer might be willing to donate services to produce a children's coloring book on bicycle safety to be distributed by the facility's staff at health fairs.

Corporate sponsorships. In exchange for name or logo visibility, many major corporations are willing to provide services and funds for a broad range of projects.

Unlike procuring many other financial resources, raising debt capital requires agreement of, and participation by, the facility's principals. The radiology administrator must prepare a well-documented proposal to the leadership, relaying the pros and cons, key terms, and project goals and outcome measures. Much of the same information will subsequently be included in the loan application.

According to Andrew Sherman, author of *Raising Capital*,[2] the loan officer must be convinced of the creditworthiness of the business and its principals before agreeing to present the loan application to the bank's loan committee, which actually decides whether to grant the loan and on what terms. Four factors determine creditworthiness:

- *Character*—the borrower's reputation and honesty.
- *Capacity*—the borrower's business experience and know-how.
- *Capital*—the borrower's ability to meet loan payments.
- *Collateral*—assets that can be liquidated in the event of default.

In addition, the loan application will call for the following:

- *A project summary*—the intended use, amount needed, repayment schedule, and collateral.
- *The borrower's history*—the facility's history, management structure, mission statement, current services, plans for growth, and key suppliers and relationships (such as managed care contractors).
- *Market research*—the facility's competition, market share, marketing communications activities, competitive advantages, and local and national trends affecting healthcare and radiology in particular.
- *Financial information*—tax returns, current balance sheet, credit references, valuations of key assets, 3-year projected cash-flow statement by month (in support of ability to repay the loan), and how debt capital will affect growth plans.
- *Supporting documentation*—organization chart; curricula vitae of principals; contracts with managed care providers, hospitals, and other key customers or vendors; leases; insurance policies; and when available, items such as annual reports, recent news articles about the facility, and newsletters.

Equity Capital—Equity capital is funds given to a business in exchange for a share of the ownership. The two most common sources of equity capital are angel investors and venture capital firms.

Angel investors are wealthy individuals who invest in businesses of high growth potential with the expectation of high returns on the investment. Most angels invest in start-up or early-stage businesses and provide funds up to $50,000; some wealthier angels may be willing to invest up to $500,000. Angels typically invest in businesses within their own geographic region and often look for opportunities that will allow them to use their substantial business experience to assist the investment business—as a consultant, mentor, or board member, for example. Angels may be attracted to an investment for reasons beyond return on investment, such as a strong affinity for the business or its principals.

These investors play a much larger role in growing businesses than might be expected. Some estimates hold that angels now provide more than 80% of total start-up and seed capital in the United States.[2] They are particularly important because many venture capital firms (see below) no longer consider investments of less than $4 million.

Attorneys or accountants are one source of referrals to an angel. However, many angels participate in nonprofit angel networks, clubs, and other "pooled" funds organizations. Matching services and venture fairs provide a structured approach to networking. Less formal networking through local service organizations (for example, Rotary International), local business organizations (for example, chambers of commerce), the state economic development agency, and healthcare organizations also may identify local angels. For more information about angel investors, contact the following:

Angel Capital Alliance
www.angelcapitalassociation.org
Active Capital
activecapital.org
Oklahoma Investment Forum
www.i2e.org

The two most relevant types of venture capital firms are small-business investment companies (SBICs) and public and private venture capital firms. SBICs are privately owned and managed, but they are licensed and regulated by the SBA. Although the SBA does not directly invest, it does guarantee at least some of the funds borrowed by the SBICs for investment. More than 400 SBICs are licensed. Like other venture capital entities, they often specialize by region, industry, or stage of business development (for example, start-up or expansion stages). Related programs focus on businesses in rural and low-income regions. A directory is available at www.sba.gov. Members of the National Association of Small Business Investment Companies can be found at www.nasbic.org.

Finally, public and private venture capital firms are usually organized as limited partnerships, which gather capital from trust funds, pension funds, insurance companies, and individual venture investors. These funds are then invested in high-growth businesses. Among the types of projects these firms might fund are major expansions (so-called third-stage financing), acquisitions or mergers, and joint ventures (see Box 4.4).

A venture capital firm funds only a half dozen deals out of thousands of business plans it sees each year. One of the most important factors in the decision is the quality of the management team: Is the team committed to the facility and the project for which funding is sought? Does it include members with a full range of business skills and experience? Are the principals confident in themselves and the facility?

Of course, financial and business factors must also meet the venture capitalist's criteria. The project should offer a 25% to 35% return on investment; the facility should have a sustainable competitive edge in its market; the venture capitalist must have some say in the project's management (for example, a seat on the board of directors);

Box 4.4 Joint Ventures: When Two Become One

One way to secure financing, specialized expertise, or both is to form a joint venture with one or more partners to carry out a project or long-term strategic objective. A second company is set up legally, as a partnership, limited liability company, or even a corporation. Each party contributes skills and resources to the venture, and if successful, each party reaps the rewards. For example, an imaging center might create a joint venture with a builder to construct a multiuse medical building, which will house the expanded center along with other practices. The builder provides construction and financial resources; the imaging center provides tenant contacts within the healthcare community, expertise on facility design, and financial resources. Another example of a joint venture may involve a hospital and physician practice working together to develop a new outpatient facility.

To be successful, a joint venture should have the following elements:

- A unified purpose for all parties involved.
- A management team committed to the project's success.
- A cooperative culture.
- Contributions from all parties that make the resulting company stronger than each party individually.
- Alignment of management and operating styles.
- Some flexibility in case changes occur in the environment, technology, or the marketplace.

and the proposal must outline how the investor will get back the investment plus return on capital within 4 to 6 years (known as the *exit strategy*).

Because competition for venture capital is so intense, the best way to have a proposal considered is through a professional referral. Investment bankers, attorneys, and accountants are other possible referral sources, as are leaders in the local business community. Other sources of leads are the National Venture Capital Association (www.nvca.org) and the National Association of Investment Companies (specializing in minority-owned businesses; www.naicvc.com).

SIDEBAR: Identifying Resources

In a thriving venture, any effort toward improvement is only as good as the resources that help formalize it. Indeed, when it comes to strategic planning in an institution, being able to identify which resources will provide the maximum outcome in results is crucial. Identifiable resources are financial, technological, and human.

Each resource offers an opportunity to expand a facility's strategic initiative from a differing vantage point. Having the correct people in place, utilizing the best in technology, and knowing which financial proposal offers maximum gain will ensure success in the marketplace. Financial, technological, and human resources can be both internal and external and offer value through learned experiences. These experiences enable a facility to forecast new strategic initiatives, develop ones that have potential, and avoid others that could inhibit growth.

Identifying Technological Resources

Assessing Current Capabilities

As Chapters 1 and 2 described, conducting baseline and needs assessments are crucial first steps in creating a strategic plan and setting goals. Such assessments, performed annually, also provide the basis for identifying the technology resources that are available to carry out the plan and meet the goals. The process becomes one of matching needs to current technology and, where gaps occur, locating alternative resources.

For example, suppose the strategic plan called for implementing a marketing communications effort to expand mammography screenings among underserved populations. Among the components planned to achieve the goal are brochures for Spanish-speaking and low-literacy readers to be distributed at health fairs, at community social gatherings, and through community agencies and primary care providers serving these target audiences. In terms of technology, the project requires computer software (and adequate computer capacity) to design the brochures and prepare them for professional printing. In this simple example, the radiology administrator should answer the following questions:

- Is the software that is now installed adequate to design the pieces to the printer's specifications?
- If yes, then does a staff member know how to use the software effectively, and is excess capacity available to carry out the project?
- If no, then what is the cost of buying, licensing, and installing the software? Are computer capacity and capabilities adequate to support it? Does a staff member know how to use it? If not, is someone available who can be trained to use it? If so, at what cost, and within what timeframe?

Depending on the answers to these questions, the radiology administrator may need to explore alternatives. For a department within a hospital or other healthcare facility, for example, design services may be available through the community affairs, marketing, public relations, or development departments. The administrator of a radiology practice with multiple offices may find the needed technology at a sister facility. A third alternative open to any radiology administrator is outsourcing to a graphic design firm or a design student from a local university.

Every goal or element of the strategic plan should be analyzed in a similar manner to assess what technology is needed, whether it now exists in the facility, and if not, where to get it. Major projects, such as offering a new modality, are likely to require both new and existing technology. The impact of new technology on existing capacity should be considered as well.

Identifying Alternative Technology Resources

Outsourcing—One alternative technology resource is outsourcing. Business process outsourcing involves hiring a business, also referred to as an *application service provider,* (ASP) to perform a specific task, such as payroll, accounts receivable, or information technology. A key advantage in outsourcing highly technical processes is the elimination of the need to purchase and support the technology, which can draw not only financial but also staff resources away from the central mission of patient care. Outsourcing also eliminates the need to invest in technology that may quickly become obsolete.

Outsourcing does have disadvantages, however. It can be difficult to manage, especially with large-scale, long-term projects. Vendor-client expectations may not be compatible. Processes with clearly defined rules and discrete boundaries, such as server maintenance, are most likely to be successfully outsourced. A well-defined contract, close collaboration between vendor and client, and careful management are essential for success.

Outsourcing is usually less expensive than performing the task internally, which is one of its most influential selling points to senior management. Pricing may be based on a flat fee for services (fixed pricing), a rate per unit of service (unit pricing), fixed pricing for basic services with additional costs for higher service levels (variable pricing), or performance with incentive payments for optimal service (performance-based pricing). No matter what type of pricing is negotiated, however, it may cost up to 10% above the contracted amount to negotiate and manage the deal.[3] Those costs include vendor selection, time and staff to educate the vendor about the facility's needs and processes, and ongoing vendor management.

Selecting an outsourcing vendor involves several phases:

1. Defining needs and expectations.
2. Identifying the potential vendors and researching their capabilities.
3. Choosing providers for the request for proposal (RFP) process.
4. Narrowing the selection based on the proposals.
5. Negotiating with the chosen vendor.

For more on vendor selection and the RFP process, see "Identifying Consulting Resources" later in the chapter.

Leasing—Another source for technology, especially equipment, is leasing. When a technology is rapidly evolving or when purchasing equipment would deplete cash flow and affect payment of day-to-day expenses, leasing is a particularly attractive option.

The advantages of leasing include the following:

- Acquiring the use of equipment without a large capital outlay.
- Gaining tax advantages by deducting lease payments as business expenses.
- Obtaining financing to purchase equipment more easily than is possible through a bank loan and at more flexible terms.
- Avoiding obsolescence.
- Leaving credit untouched, for potential use on other projects.

Leasing also has disadvantages, of course:

- Lack of ownership; the equipment is not a facility asset and must be purchased (or the lease extended) on the lease's expiration.

- Substantial costs in finance charges that will make leasing a more costly option than purchasing from cash flow.
- The need to make lease payments even if equipment is no longer in use, or to pay a penalty to terminate the lease.

As with all contracts, the radiology administrator should carefully review the lease agreement, in consultation with the CFO and attorney, and negotiate the best terms possible before signing. In particular, the administrator should scrutinize the cancellation policy, warranty and maintenance terms, and penalties and fees beyond the monthly payments. Also, for rapidly evolving technology, it is advantageous to negotiate a modern-equipment substitution clause that allows the facility to update before the end of the lease, or to consider a shorter lease term than standard (despite potentially higher monthly payments).

Sharing—In some communities, two or more radiology departments in competing hospitals share ownership and use of a mobile PET unit. This sharing allows each facility to offer a new modality to their patients at a lower capital expenditure and operating cost, without expensive downtime. For such a major piece of equipment, of course, a joint venture or other contractual arrangement is necessary.

Sharing technology may also be as straightforward as several departments within a facility allocating funds from their budgets to purchase one color printer, scanner, or other modest piece of specialized equipment for all to use. This sharing may be particularly attractive for equipment that is used only occasionally but that contributes substantially to achieving one or more goals. Although such an arrangement can be less formal than that required to jointly own a PET unit, it is nevertheless wise to have a written understanding about where the device will be housed, who will be responsible for such things as supplies and maintenance, and how use will be scheduled.

Identifying Human Resources

Some goals may actually reduce the level of human resource use; an example is shortening patient check-in time by eliminating one step in the process. More commonly, achieving goals and carrying out a strategic plan will require staff time and expertise, even if the ultimate result is increased productivity and reduction of FTEs. It is a rare facility that has excess staffing capacity. It is essential to set priorities among the goals and between new projects and ongoing tasks; it is also necessary to analyze what skills, knowledge, and time commitment will be required. Based on this assessment, the radiology administrator is ready to identify the human resources—within the organization and beyond—necessary to make things happen.

Analyzing Internal Human Resources

An investment in personnel evaluation will offer extensive insight into the "rising stars" within the organization. Carrying out a successful strategic plan is a clear opportunity to invest in these staff members.

Rising stars are individuals who are successful because they are highly motivated, well compensated, and happy with their jobs. Many rising stars have entrepreneurial thought processes or consider themselves to be entrepreneurs, and they thrive in an environment that offers freedom, flexibility, and openness. Because of their success and sense of belonging, these individuals are less likely to leave and more dedicated to their work. They communicate to others that they are satisfied with their job.

The most common motivators for rising stars are the challenges and responsibilities that come with their jobs. The more complex the challenge, the happier these employees are. Additional experiences and leadership opportunities are the driving forces of these individuals. They are ideal candidates to champion a project, especially if their input was sought during the initial planning process, thus giving them an early sense of project ownership.

"Work-in-progress" staff members are the most abundant category in the workplace. Their number makes them a more formidable force to reckon with than other workers, as well as essential allies to ensure the success of the strategic plan. These individuals are moldable and usually can be drawn into supporting goals and plans. Work-in-progress staff members have the potential to become rising stars and will work harder if what they believe in is perceived as credibile in terms of department and facility goals.

Having the insight to identify the rising stars is important, but equally important is the ability to identify the "falling stars," personnel who have lost their vision, drive, and motivation. Although in comparison with rising stars they are more numerous and more tedious to work with, and the organization expends a disproportionate amount of energy on them they can offer insight into where work needs to be done. In particular, their often pessimistic view of why something should not succeed can provide valuable information that can be used to gain unified support for planned projects and goals.

The new goals and plans present an opportunity to change, mold, and nurture these individuals, some of whom may be groomed to become rising stars. Even employees who are good at their work tasks while merely plodding through the day can effectively carry out aspects of strategic initiatives. And even if falling stars lack rising star qualities, they often have valuable characteristics that can help hold a strategic plan together. When they are given guidance and direction, and when they understand the causes and effects of their contribution to the project, these employees may become motivated. A "buy-in" approach to these individuals often yields good results. In contrast, falling stars who fail to respond to the opportunities posed by new goals and projects may become a liability, and the wise decision for both employer and employee is to let them go.

To identify the types of employees the facility has to work with and to match their skills to the needs of a project, start with the performance review process and personnel records. The facility's human resource staff should be able to facilitate this task, as will creating a workforce profile. The profile includes data related to current staff members on job classification and section, skills, age and gender, experience, character, scheduling flexibility, and potential for advancement.

Whenever possible, staff members should be involved in discussions about human resource utilization to achieve goals. Individuals who have input in the planning stage may be eager to champion a project. Staff members who are responsible for tasks that will be directly affected by a goal may be in the best position to devise staff responsibilities to achieve it. For example, if the goal is to reduce patient check-in time, the reception staff and technologists are familiar with the current process and may offer suggestions and take responsibility for changing traffic flow or revising forms.

The strategic plan may offer chances for career advancement and cross-training incentives. These opportunities can be important to rising star staff members and may be the incentive needed by work-in-progress employees to become more motivated. In implementing improvements, altering a service line, or modifying services, it is important to ask whether the expected result can be handled with current staffing levels and expertise. If a service line's current staff cannot take on the task, can someone be transferred or cross-trained to achieve the goal? For example, if a facility wants to expand its use of abdominal CT scanning in place of intravenous pyelography, it may be necessary to transfer staff from general radiology to CT and provide additional training to handle the shifting patient load.

New responsibilities can reignite the fire in some employees and help with recruitment and retention. If the plan attempts to promote or market services, find those individuals who do it best. If the goal is to increase volume in a particular imaging modality, determine who has the most appropriate skill sets to carry it out.

Using cross-trained individuals can produce a better return on investment than hiring additional staff or outsourcing. It can also demonstrate to staff members that they are held in a high regard and are entrusted to be a significant part of the facility's growth and success.

Identifying Alternative Human Resources: Temporary Staffing and Outsourcing

When the achievement of goals calls for significant increases in staff hours (FTEs) or for skills unavailable in existing staff, the radiology administrator can consider at least two alternatives: temporary staffing and outsourcing. (Outsourcing was discussed earlier in is chapter.)

Many regions are facing a shortage of healthcare workers, including radiology technologists, so temporary workers are a familiar feature in most settings. The ability to hire a skilled worker for a limited time makes temporary hiring a worthwhile staffing alternative in carrying out one-time projects of limited scope and timeframe.

Hiring temporary workers offers a number of advantages:

- Helping meet short-term demands of special projects or workload fluctuations.
- Providing an opportunity to evaluate workers without a long-term commitment.
- Providing access to workers with specialized skills.
- Giving skilled workers flexibility and allowing them to remain in the workforce, rather than leaving, because they are unable or unwilling to work full-time.
- Providing a cost-effective option, especially for jobs lasting less than 6 months, when compared with salary and benefits for a full-time employee.

Among the disadvantages of hiring temporary workers are the following:

- Need for training, at least about facility-specific processes and organizational hierarchy, which lessens productivity of both the temporary worker and the individual providing the training.
- Lack of continuity when the temporary worker leaves.
- Potential morale issues, especially for workers on long temporary assignments and temporary workers who do not receive benefits from their agency employer comparable to those of permanent staff.

- Potential safety issues, as the frequency and severity of on-the-job injuries have been found to be higher among temporary workers than permanent staff.[4]
- Legal concerns over the independent contractor status of temporary workers, especially those on long-term assignment

Large radiology departments within multiservice healthcare facilities or imaging centers with several locations may have access to PRN (*pro re nata,* or "as-needed") technologists. PRN pools frequently draw on former permanent employees who now provide their services intermittently as independent contractors, reducing the time needed for orientation and facility-specific training.

A staffing agency is a more widely available source of temporary workers. The caliber of the agency will be reflected in the caliber of its workers, so the radiology administrator should take time to find a reputable, reliable firm. The process for locating a staffing agency is much the same as for finding other vendors. Getting referrals from colleagues and finding names in the local Yellow Pages are useful. Preliminary research can be carried out by viewing the companies' Web sites, calling the Better Business Bureau to see if complaints have been filed, and asking colleagues for information and referrals. Questions to ask key staffing agency personnel include the following:

- If the agency does not specialize in healthcare, what proportion of its clients or placements are in the healthcare industry?
- How does the agency recruit and retain its workforce?
- How are workers screened? How does the agency verify licensing, credentials, and so on?
- What benefits does the agency provide to its workers? Does it carry workers' compensation insurance?
- Is the agency a member of the American Staff Association or another professional organization? To which local business organizations do its staffing personnel belong?
- Can the agency supply references?

As with other staffing resources, the more clearly the radiology administrator describes to the agency the job to be performed and the skills needed, the greater the likelihood of finding a qualified temporary worker with the first placement.

Identifying Consulting Resources

Consultants range from graphic designers to management consultants. Despite their diversity, they share a number of characteristics, many of which offer special advantages to their clients. First, consultants present an "outside, looking in" approach to problem solving and planning. They can be objective in evaluating alternatives, the potential for success, and the reasons for failure. Second, they have knowledge and insight gained from working on similar projects; they can help the radiology administrator learn from the mistakes of others and gain from their best practices. Third, consultants can provide a set of specialized or advanced skills not available within the facility's staff.

Determining the scope of the project and the expertise needed are crucial first steps that will influence not only the final selection of consultants but also the extent of the selection process. For one-time or small-scale projects or projects requiring a unique skill set with limited availability of local experts, interviewing one consultant may be adequate and the most productive method. Asking colleagues or vendors for referrals and consulting the local Yellow Pages can provide leads to qualified consultants. Another resource is professional associations for consultants:

Independent Computer Consultants Association

www.icca.org

Association of Management Consulting Firms

www.amcf.org

Association of Professional Consultants

www.consultapc.org

Institute of Management Consultants USA

www.imcusa.org

Radiology administrators who work within large hospitals or healthcare facilities may have access to a prequalified pool of consultants through the purchasing or human resources department. After reviewing the list and selecting a small group of qualified consultants, the administrator contacts each one, explains the scope of the project, and establishes the consultant's interest and availability. The third step involves asking for a general description of how the consultant would approach the project and perhaps scheduling an interview. After selecting one finalist, that consultant is asked to submit a more detailed project description with costs. If negotiations fail to reach agreement on the scope of the project or costs, the radiology administrator approaches the second-choice consultant for details and costs.

If a prequalified pool is not available or a single consultant cannot be identified for a simple project, the request for qualifications (RFQ) process can help locate viable candidates. This process includes the following steps:

1. *Announcing the availability of an RFQ.* An advertisement may be placed in local newspapers, business and professional publications and Web sites, and even on the facility's Web site, as well as being sent to firms that represent possible candidates. The notice announces that the facility is seeking a consultant, briefly describes the project, and provides information for requesting an RFQ form.
2. *Sending the RFQ.* Consultants who respond to the advertisement receive the RFQ, which asks for contact information, key personnel information, a statement of qualifications for the project, availability, a client or project list, and references.
3. *Ranking the candidates.* Based on the RFQ response, the candidates are ranked in terms of their suitability for the project. The top one to three candidates (depending on time, scope of the project, and strength of the candidate pool) receive additional scrutiny, including reference checks and possibly telephone or in-person interviews.
4. *Selecting the candidate.* One candidate is selected from the finalists, and the process then becomes the same as selecting from a prequalified pool, as described above.

For larger projects or ones that are likely to continue for months or even years, the radiology administrator may want to use the RFP process, alone or in conjunction with the RFQ process. The RFP may be advertised as the RFQ is, be mailed to a large group of consultants, or be sent to a select pool of candidates. It is wise to keep the number distributed to a manageable level. Although it may seem a good idea to get as many proposals as possible, reviewing each proposal can be time-consuming. In addition, qualified consultants may hesitate to respond if they see the process as a "fishing expedition" or a search that lacks focus.

Consultants who express a willingness to submit a proposal receive the RFP. Complex projects, such as installing PACS or conducting renovations, may call for an informal preproposal conference at which all interested consultants can ask questions, view the facility, and collect additional documents (such as facility brochures) to help them prepare a relevant, realistic proposal. Once all the proposals have been received, each must be reviewed according to specific criteria relevant to the project. A preliminary ranking should result in the selection of one to three consultants for in-person interviews. When a finalist has been selected, the process continues as described above.

No matter what the scope of the project is or what process is used to select a consultant, certain information is crucial to a successful project and working relationship:

- The consultant's experience and its relevance to the project.
- The consultant's work style (for example, willingness to make suggestions and level of collaboration).
- Deliverables to expect (for example, interim and final reports, site plans, project specifications, and volume growth).
- Procedural details (consultant staff assigned to the project, the progress reporting process, the timeline, facility staff needed, and termination).
- Financial details (total costs, fee breakdown and structure, payment schedule, and ownership of the final product).

Conclusion

Creating a successful strategic plan and completing set goals are fundamental to ensuring the success and growth of a facility. Yet no plan can be carried out without expending resources, including financial, technological, and human resources. Identifying the resources that will be available to meet goals and achieve the plan becomes critical to a facility's accomplishments.

Strategic initiatives can become successful ventures if a facility uses the correct financial resources. Although plans to acquire capital equipment will likely call for a financial commitment beyond the facility's balance sheet, the radiology administrator in a well-run institution will often find the financial resources to carry out other plans in cash reserves, profits, revenue growth, and budget savings.

The technological resources of a facility are an important factor in the success of a strategic plan and, if needed, in attracting new business. Conducting baseline and needs assessments are crucial steps in creating a strategic plan and setting goals. Such assessments, performed annually, also provide the basis for identifying the technology resources that are available to carry out the plan and meet the goals. The process involves matching needs to current applicable technology.

Identifying financial and technological resources is extremely important, but incorporation of the human factor also is crucial. Achieving goals and carrying out a strategic plan usually requires staff time and expertise. In goal achievement, setting priorities among the goals in both new projects and ongoing tasks is essential, as is analyzing the skills, knowledge, and time commitment required. Based on this assessment, the radiology administrator can identify the human resources—within the organization and beyond—needed to make things happen.

Utilizing the facility's financial, technological, and human resources and analyzing its past to project the progress in the future is a task worth undertaking.

References

1. Sferrella SM, Allen ML, Reitter MS, eds. *Financial Management in Radiology.* Sudbury, MA: American Healthcare Radiology Administrators; 2004.

2. Sherman AJ. *Raising Capital: Get the Money You Need to Grow Your Business.* 2nd ed. New York, NY: American Management Association; 2005.

3. Overby S. The ABCs of outsourcing. Available at: http://www.cio.com/article/ 118100/The_ABCs_of_Outsourcing. Accessed July 27, 2007.

4. Schaefer P. The pros and cons of hiring a temp. Available at: http://www. businessknowhow.com/manage/hire-temp.htm. Accessed January 4, 2007.

Chapter 5

Research to Strategy: Assessing the External and Internal Environments

Elsa Ozuna-Richards

This chapter focuses on a critical component of strategic planning—market research. A thorough understanding of the market is crucial to the strategic process. Research, as the prelude to strategic planning, supports the decision-making processes and financial investments involved in the growth of a radiology facility. This chapter introduces a process for evaluating market characteristics of both the internal environment and the external environment (including the customers and competitors).

Long gone are the days of considering the "radiology business" simply as "a practice." In today's competitive environment, the radiology facility must operate on solid business principles involving market research, strategic planning, strategic marketing, customer retention, value propositions, technology offerings, competitive comparisons, and financial management. Without knowledge of the market and specific customer demands, the radiology facility will be ineffective in delivering value to its customers and differentiating itself from competitors.

Although many individuals in the radiology service industry may feel they know their customers, market research can provide a detailed perspective on the attitudes, behaviors, wants, and specific needs of the customer. It provides a better understanding about the services and goods in which the customer is interested. With today's competitive market and the costs associated with providing leading-edge technology, consumer research is an important foundation for the strategic process.

The radiology industry is a highly competitive environment, which requires a true gauge of the competition. If facilities assess their competitors with the same level of interest and detail as they evaluate their customers, they are likely to gain a comprehensive perspective of market deficits in service and delivery. This knowledge contributes to their ability to tailor service programs to meet specific needs and thus bring greater value to the customer.

Evaluating competitors through the eyes of the customer is the litmus test for service performance. Facilities should not rely on intuition or past experiences to determine their strengths and weaknesses. They should allow customers to communicate their perspectives. Conducting customer surveys pinpoints the service characteristics of key competitors that customers value.

Understanding the internal environment and culture helps a business tweak (or totally reconstruct) customer service benchmarks and parameters. If service promises cannot be delivered, brand equity is lost. Making workflow conducive to optimal service delivery improves customer attitudes and strengthens brand loyalty.

Economic and political influences are external forces that may affect the success of a facility. Understanding the intricacies of the political arena is vital to a healthcare company's livelihood. Other elements of the external environment that can directly affect the operation and finances of a radiology facility are businesses the facility works with, such as the manufacturing firms and suppliers that control equipment, supplies, and service costs.

Definitions

Market research entails gaining information about the people in a geographic area. This information can include demographics, population by segments, economic status, growth trends, and education levels. Market research expands that information and involves learning more about attitudes, perceptions, needs, and wants of the people within a defined target market.

Market informatics can be gleaned using two methods: primary research and secondary research. Methodology varies depending on the problem. *Primary research* involves collecting data about the customer by way of surveys, personal interviews, observation, and focus groups. *Secondary research* is conducted using studies that have already been performed and published, such as governmental studies, technologic publications, political issues, legislation, business reports, and trade publications.

Primary data can be collected by qualitative or quantitative research methods. *Qualitative research* involves obtaining a more subjective perspective about beliefs, perceptions, values, and behavior. This research deals with the "why" in human behavior. The information is gathered through techniques that are less structured, though precise in regard to research objectives. Qualitative techniques allow for more open-ended questioning to gain a deeper perspective on customers.

Quantitative research is based on collecting statistical data through questionnaires and surveys to assess the opinions of a larger population base. Statistical data are used to measure relationships among the various data elements or objectives. Because of the larger sampling size, this research technique can be used as a foundation for projecting and measuring.

Market Research Process

The prospect of a long and tedious process is not appealing to busy professionals. Figure 5.1 provides a simple overview of any research process. Whether conducting a full market assessment (comprehensive demographics, customer surveys, and competitive analysis) or simply one component of the assessment, it is important to focus clearly on the objectives. Keeping processes simple is important. This diagram organizes the process into three areas: the event, the preparation, and the research function.

Internal and External Environments

Internal Environment

Internal assessments should be conducted in a two-prong approach. First, begin at the corporate level with the key stakeholders. Second, conduct staff interviews and perform a detailed workflow assessment. The work processes should be designed to meet the demands and needs of each customer segment. The latter involves

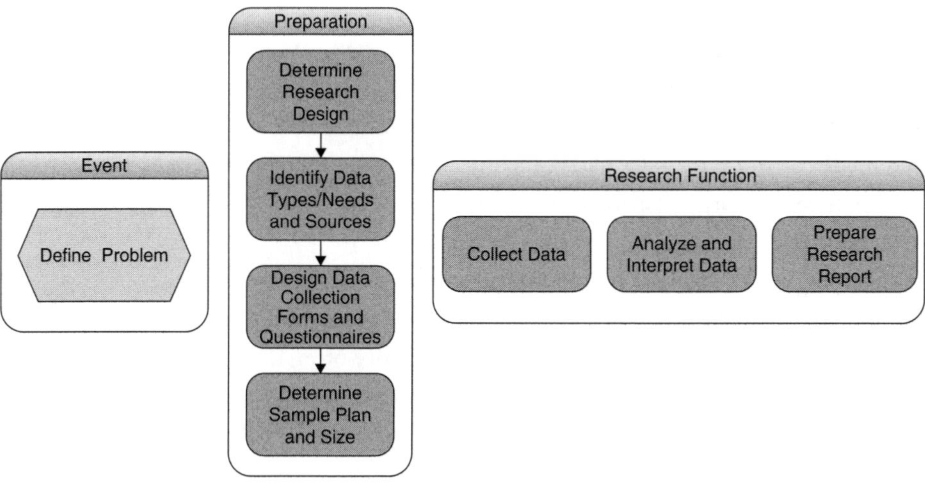

Figure 5.1 Overview of the research process.

reengineering processes to increase operational efficiency, improve performance quality, and reduce costs.

Starting at the Top—Vision and direction come from the top. Skilled leadership with an entrepreneurial sense is necessary to position and differentiate a radiology facility from its competitors. The assessment begins by gaining the key stakeholders' perspective about their own business, position in the market, and vision for the future. Are the owners of the facility committed to developing a strategy that brings value to their customers?

Research begins at the top of the organization with some fundamentals such as a preliminary SWOT (strengths, weaknesses, opportunities, and threats) analysis. Participants should identify and prioritize elements in each of the four areas. It is best to work with a facilitator who can bring objectivity into the discussion. This exercise will provide a solid foundation to, and some excellent insight into, the operations of the business. A comprehensive SWOT analysis will be developed as the research progresses.

Operational Workflow—Various approaches are possible in the evaluation and improvement of business processes and the leveraging of current resources (labor and equipment). The workflow assessment requires evaluating current processes, reengineering work processes to improve operational efficiency, goal setting (setting service performance goals), and testing outcomes (metrics). Every aspect of the internal environment must be scrutinized for obstacles that deter efficient work flow.

Something as simple as "attaching yourself to the requisition" provides valuable information about the operations and environment and identifies where inefficiencies exist. By walking through every process in the organization, service levels are elevated and cycle times for each department are improved when the focus is shifted to reducing the number of steps and improving the quality of service delivery to each customer segment. If internal resources are not available for this type of assessment, an outside consultant can be used to bring a nonbiased perspective in order to tweak or reengineer the organization's processes.

Regular employee training ensures that staff is trained well and the error rate is minimized. Service outcomes become more predictable and more error-free. Costs are reduced because errors are minimized and, more often than not, fewer hands are required to accomplish tasks. The facility attains a stronger competitive position. The workflow assessment should also be performed in collaboration with staff members to fully secure their buy-in to the process and ensure that each individual understands his or her role and impact on a successful outcome.

External Environment

It is important to understand external market dynamics that affect the facility's ability to meet its business objectives and thrive. These dynamics include customers, competitors, hospital systems, suppliers, technologic advancements, and legislation affecting operations. Each of these elements provides critical information regarding trends, perceptions, needs, and purchasing drivers that are vital components of the decision-making and planning processes.

The healthcare customer can be segmented into the referring source (referring group practice), patient (including family members and prospective patients), hospital/healthcare system, payor, and supplier/vendor. Each segment has its own set of needs, perceptions, and basis for brand loyalty. It is important to view an organization through the eyes of each of its customers.

Refraining from making personal assumptions when profiling customers allows for a fresh perspective and opens the opportunity for exploring better ways to deliver value to each segment. By identifying the current needs, a facility can determine how each customer defines value, where each customer is going to get its current needs met, and how the facility's infrastructure can be adapted to excel at meeting those needs.

The most obvious radiology customers are referring physicians and staff, patients, payors and health networks, hospital systems, and internal customers (staff members). The market analysis should focus on obtaining the customers' perspectives about their interactions with the radiology facility or competing providers. By reaffirmings basic needs, understanding emotional triggers, and identifying which service offerings are perceived to provide value, the radiology facility can distinguish elements of the purchasing behavior to which service offerings can be tailored. Doing so also identifies other opportunities.

The Patient as Customer—Every customer segment should be evaluated in each of the following categories:

- *Demographics.* In each specific area, who makes up the target market? How does each group access healthcare services, and what is the normal use of healthcare services for each group?
- *Psychographics and sociographics.* What are the target market's lifestyle attitudes, social status, and religion? How do these variables affect the selection of a radiology provider? Which elements are involved in making a decision about health service providers? How does each group define value with regard to healthcare and imaging services?

- *Economic status.* How does the overall economic status affect the utilization of health services? Does economic status affect the decision of healthcare providers in the target market?
- *Health status.* How healthy is the target market, and what are the key health status indicators? What type of diagnostic services will address the key health indicators?

Demographics—Radiology practices are data rich. The typical radiology information systems offer management reports with a wealth of information about the patient customer. Almost everything that needs to be known about the patient customer resides in the database. It is an excellent tool for obtaining a comprehensive view of the type of customer that is driving growth.

Research elements should include age, education, gender, race, ethnicity, patient history, provisional diagnosis, and actual diagnosis broken out by zip code or specific area. What are the trends or growth areas? If particular geographic areas have higher health risks or segmented clusters of population, expansion in those areas should respond to the specific needs of that area.

Psychographics and Sociographics—Recognizing what drives the purchasing behavior of the target segments determines how market services should be packaged and delivered. Will cultural differences, values, religion, or social status come into play with regard to services offered and delivery? How many amenities will be required to develop brand loyalty and increase brand equity in a particular market?

Economic Status—Is there healthy economic development in the areas in which patients reside or work? Are new businesses flocking to the area? Where, geographically, is the growth? How long is it projected to last? Are people employed and represented by health insurance? What are the current and projected forecasts for the housing market? What kinds of health plans represent the community? The answers to these questions affect whether your facility will continue to grow in the environment and where future expansion may be required to meet the needs of the patient population.

Health Status—Are there any health indicators that affect the patients' well-being? If there are distinctive health issues and trends in the target market, equipment planning can meet the specific diagnostic needs. State and local agencies can provide this information. Large healthcare organizations, such as hospitals and health systems, are also excellent resources. Evaluating the facility's own management reports to identify ICD9 trends provides the most immediate information.

The Referring Physician as Customer

Demographics—In the United States, the average number of physicians in a county is 169.7 per 100,000, or approximately 1.57 per 1,000. Physicians and surgeons held about 567,000 jobs in 2004; approximately 1 out of 7 was self-employed and not incorporated. Approximately 60% of salaried physicians and surgeons were in an office of physicians, and 16% were employed by private hospitals. (According to the US Department of Labor, Bureau of Labor Statistics, office-based physicians include all MDs and DOs who report that 80% or more of their work is in the office setting.) Others practiced in federal, state, and local governments, including hospitals, colleges, universities, and professional schools, as well as in outpatient care centers. According to the American Medical Association, in 2003, approximately 2 out 5 physicians were in primary care, but not in a subspecialty of primary care (Table 5.1).[1]

Individual markets may have very different physician and specialist populations. Before investing in high-cost equipment, it is important to get a detailed assessment of the physician population in a target market. Doing so involves mapping specialists geographically to identify where the physician/specialist pockets are located, thus indicating potential demand for services, high-end technology, and diagnostic facilities.

Where is the physician population moving? If the area is developing and expanding, family practice physicians will arrive in the area very soon. Geographic shifts in the general population and physician infiltration have obvious effects on the demand

Table 5.1 Percentage Distribution of Physicians

	Percent
Total	100.0
Primary care	40.8
Family medicine and general practice	12.8
Internal medicine	15.1
Obstetrics and gynecology	5.3
Pediatrics	7.6
Specialties	59.2
Anesthesiology	5.4
Psychiatry	5.4
Surgical specialties, selected	14.6
All other specialties	33.9

Source: American Medical Association, *Physician Characteristics and Distribution in the US*, 2005.

for diagnostic imaging. Tracking growth projections and trends is vital to effective strategic planning. Growth in the economy is a sure indication of good things to come with regard to growth in a community.

Psychographics and Sociographics—What drives purchasing behavior in specific markets? Each market is distinct, and radiology facilities should determine what drives physician referrals in their markets. Are these referrals based solely on managed care networks, proximity to radiology providers, and customer service delivery (prompt appointments and reports), or does the radiologists' expertise affect the referrals?

Several market studies have shown that managed care (or health plans) is not always the key driver in securing referrals. In many markets that seem to be driven by managed care, in an even playing field (multiple radiology providers on a network), customer service performance ultimately drives the referral. Factors include the radiologists' responsiveness, quick report turnaround, prompt appointments, and staff friendliness.

Radiology providers should identify service expectations and then work to exceed them. Regardless of how restrictive a managed care market is, radiology providers should optimize their abilities to develop a "customer-centric" environment. In the most restrictive market, the referring sources will send patients to the participating provider when required. However, they send other referrals to facilities where the service delivery meets their needs. These referrals should be cultivated. One method is to identify key areas where the organization's workflow is not conducive to key referring offices.

> *Example: A urologic surgeon's office was having difficulty with the service from its radiology provider. The radiology provider would often call the office requesting laboratory test results for patients referred for procedures such as CT scans and intravenous pyelography. The nurses were busy seeing patients and could not respond to the calls until their lunch breaks. By that time, the radiology patients had been rescheduled for their radiology examinations because of the missing results. The office repeatedly requested that the radiology provider call the primary care physician or laboratory for the results. Because most of their patients were sent as referrals, the urologic surgeon's office did not have a patient record until the patient's workup was completed and the office received records from the primary care physician.*

This situation affected how soon patients could be seen by the urologic surgeon. It was created by ineffective communication and caused the urologic surgeon to send many referrals to a competing radiologic facility.

Referring office staff are always interested in providing input to improve their ability to take care of their patients' needs. The researcher should work closely with both the staff members of the radiology facility and the referring staff members to troubleshoot difficulties in service delivery. Alternatives to the current flow should be sought in order to improve the ease and time of service delivery. This exercise can greatly strengthen customer loyalty.

The Competition—It is important to maintain a clear vision of current competitors in the market, in addition to potential competitors. Anticipating changes in the competitive landscape strengthens a facility's ability to sustain a competitive edge.

Most service providers constantly monitor their competitors' tactical marketing events but fail to understand strategic vulnerabilities and key strengths. Customers are the best resource for determining the optimal service offering and delivery methods. Best practices recognize, improve on, and offer better solutions or services than their competitors. Doing so is what differentiates one competitor from another.

Conducting a competitive analysis consists of many elements. First, an organization should localize all competitors on the radar and profile each of them. Questions about the competitors to answer include, but are not limited to, the following:

- Where are the competitors located geographically, and which market niches do they serve?
- What are the competitors' strengths and weaknesses?
- What are the customers' perceptions and attitudes regarding the competing brands?
- How extensive are the competitors' service offerings?
- How do the competitors position themselves? In other words, how does the facility's market define its services and customer service relative to its competitors? (Is the facility regarded as "the high-tech radiology provider," "the friendly-service provider," or "the provider with a location on every corner"?)
- Do the competitors service a specific niche market (for example, open MRI or CT body scanning)?
- What are the future projections for the competitors' market niches?
- Are the competitors just a step ahead of the facility or always a step behind?
- What is each competitor's market share?

The competitors' strengths and weaknesses should be evaluated in relationship to the facility. Defining competitive advantages, as well as disadvantages, provides a realistic viewpoint and increases the potential for optimizing positioning strategies. Doing so requires the utmost objectivity.

Researching the competition should be conducted using primary and secondary research methods. Marketing materials, Web sites, positioning statements, and service offerings should be evaluated. "Mystery shopping" can be used to learn about competitors, as can calling competing sites to evaluate customer service standards. The researcher can identify advantages and disadvantages in each component of the process, such as prompt answering of phones, accessible appointment times, friendliness, and knowledgeable staff.

Any news stories, radiologists' articles, and other publications released by competing facilities should be reviewed to track competitors closely. Surveys should ask a simple question: What are your key radiology provider's strongest attributes? The answers should indicate how each competitor is perceived. They also will help with branding. What differentiating quality would the facility like to etch in the customer's mind?

Tackling the Research Process

Whether in launching a new facility or evaluating a market to determine customer satisfaction, gaining the customers' perspective requires asking questions. What is the question or problem the research is attempting to answer? A well-thought-out problem provides clear focus to the project and establishes the objectives for the marketing research.

Sample Study: A radiology group is planning to open a facility in a new market. The group has no brand recognition in this market and therefore does not have any established referral relationships. The group has made some basic assumptions about the market but has virtually no concrete data regarding the market's potential. Simply put, the radiology group would like to know the following:

1. *Does the market need a new facility?*
2. *If a new facility is needed, what services should it offer?*
3. *Will referring physicians send patients to the new facility?*
4. *Who is now serving these needs?*

Specific information is needed to proceed with the planning of the new facility:

- Market research (including general demographics, growth trends, and physician population).
- Perspective on the market's key referral drivers and service demands.
- An understanding of referring sources' relationships with current service providers.
- Information regarding customer satisfaction with current providers.

- Assessment of the competition and their current market penetration (current brand loyalty).
- Indications regarding barriers to entry in the market.
- Potential "physician champions" in the market.
- Information on a perceived need for a new diagnostic imaging facility.
- Indications on whether physicians will refer patients to the new facility.

Research Preparation

What is the most effective way to obtain information? Gathering information is especially problematic in the medical field, where referring offices are extremely busy. Beyond the receptionist, people strictly screen calls, and appointments are slotted for sick people only. It may seem that the only way to get feedback from referring physicians is to tackle them in the parking lot!

After the information needs have been identified, research techniques are evaluated for their effectiveness in obtaining the necessary information. More than one technique may be needed to obtain critical market information. Seeking help to develop the best method may be wise if the process seems overwhelming.

Sample Study: For this assessment, the strategic planning team decided that planting a new facility in a new market requires primary and secondary research. It was determined that a qualitative survey of the potential referring sources would best address the primary research requirement.

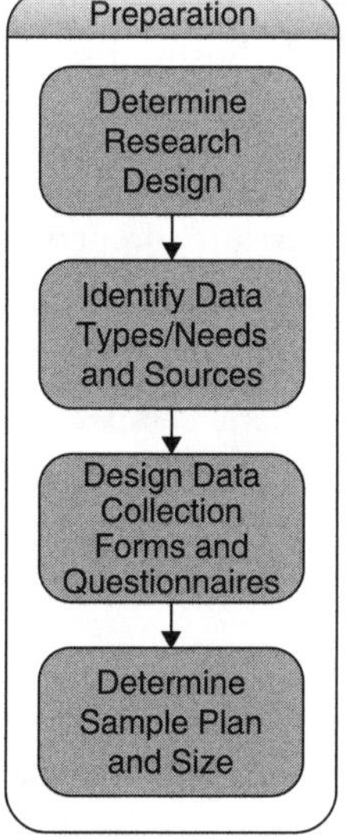

Figure 5.2 Research preparation.

Primary research techniques include the following:

- Face-to-face interviews.
- Mail, telephone, and e-mail surveys.
- Direct observation, focus groups, or both.

At this point it is important to define the metrics and parameters to measure the data and findings. The assessment also requires a full competitive analysis with some perspective about the utilization demands in the market.

Secondary research requires the following information:

- Demographics, the market's managed care infiltration, and health plan presence.
- The physician population, specialty breakout, and complete physician listing with location and contact information.
- Articles about the healthcare environment.
- Research on competitors' company profiles.
- Information about the competitors' community involvement.

The internal assessment will include assessments of areas such as financing, operational infrastructure, and workflow analysis.

Identifying Data Needs and Sources

The referring physicians, their staff, and health plan representatives in the market are primary resources for the information necessary to understand the needs of the community. Other sources with a wealth of information on health imaging needs, growth, and market trends include hospital systems, suppliers, business contacts, and business developers.

These groups can also identify barriers to entry in the market. They are excellent resources for information regarding current brand loyalty (referral relationships), and they may provide information on relationships that need to be cultivated. Business contacts provide an excellent perspective about the changes in healthcare players and trends in the commercial realty market. Information sources should be included when conducting market research. All perspectives should be considered for the planning phase.

> *Sample Study: A new facility is initially proposed as an MRI, CT, and mammography facility. Is this what is really needed in the market? Preliminary secondary research reveals that the proposed site is adjacent to a cluster of primary care physicians*

and three key specialist groups—pulmonary, orthopedics, and urologic. The target area is predicted to encompass a 6-mile radius, which also includes an excellent referring physician population.

Survey questions should deal with the following information needs:

- What drives the physicians' decision to send patients to one radiology facility over a competing facility?
- What do these physicians need with regard to imaging services?
- What distinctive referral loyalties exist?
- Is there strong brand loyalty among the "patient" customers?
- Who are the competitors, and what is their market share?
- Are there barriers to entry in the market? What are they?
- Who are the potential "physician champions" in the market?
- Is there a perceived need for a new diagnostic imaging facility?
- Will the physicians refer patients to the new facility for the proposed services?

The targeted respondents should include key personnel with decision-making responsibility for referrals to a radiology facility. These individuals typically understand the health plan requirements, know physicians' preferences, and consider the patients' needs when scheduling for diagnostic services. Physicians are difficult to reach; contacting and obtaining responses from support staff is easier and informative.

Designing Data Collection

Designing an effective survey tool is critical to obtaining the most useful information. Questions must be asked in such a way as to obtain the precise information needed. Whether the primary research uses quantitative or qualitative methodology, critical attention must be paid to the questions, which should be simple and specific.

Although in-house research can yield good information, it is often advantageous to hire an outside source for surveys. Doing so keeps objectivity in the process and allows experts to optimize time with the respondents. There are many reputable and cost-effective sources.

Sample Study: Because the data are qualitative, the team uses a survey design that includes some open-ended questions. The tool offers yes/no questions and involves a rating system to evaluate customer satisfaction. It allows for a quick, succinct survey that easily correlates with the objectives. These questions will make coding responses and interpretation easier.

Determining Sample Plan and Study Size

Techniques exist for calculating sample sizes required to estimate statistical inferences with a high level of precision. Large quantitative studies require well-defined sample sizes. Several factors are taken into consideration to achieve the correct sample size to draw accurate conclusions. Obviously, the larger the sample size, the greater the confidence that the responses truly reflect the target group.

In a qualitative study, which is primarily what a radiology facility would use for market research, there is no precise formula. Preferably, such elements as size of the market, population density, physician population, and hospital population within a targeted area are included in the determination. Even with no precise formula for qualitative studies, the criteria for targeting respondents should be carefully evaluated and designed. The sample size should be sufficient to offer a solid confidence level for strategic decisions.

Collecting the Data

Good data collection practices should be maintained throughout the study. Quality control in the collection procedures maintains integrity in the outcome of the results. These simple procedures should be followed:

- Ensure a well-defined sampling process (for example, a well-defined script and questions).
- Keep the data in chronological order.
- Document *all* comments.
- Perform data verification and cleaning (respondents' commentary, incomplete surveys, and so on).
- Develop a method for coding the responses. (This is necessary for accurate interpretation and deals with applying standardized labels, values, and rating formats to the various data elements to ensure proper measurement.)
- Report all responses, including nonresponses.
- Develop a method for transforming the data into useful information.

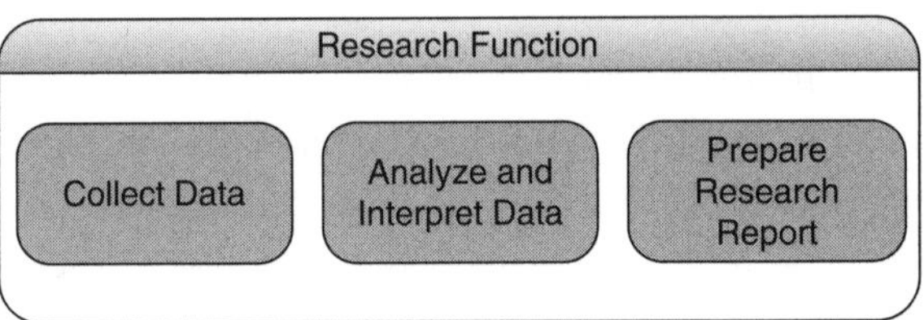

Figure 5.3 Organizing and collecting data.

Analysis and Interpretation

The information gathered from a market assessment should allow for better-informed strategic decision making. The data should identify growth opportunities, strategic vulnerabilities (problems or areas for improvement), customer needs and demands, and brand recognition or perception.

To truly maintain a competitive edge, an outside agency can be used to help ensure a nonbiased interpretation of the information, which is valuable for decision making. Stakeholders should insist on maintaining objectivity in all decision making. Objectivity in the interpretation and analysis phase also improves a facility's ability to widen its view.

The process in smaller qualitative studies includes correlating all responses and respondent commentary to questions. Responses are then tabulated to provide an accurate depiction of the environment and customers' perceptions. Although information is anecdotal, collectively it should provide actionable recommendations to decision makers. The responses, in combination with internal corporate information, should provide an excellent foundation for progressing to the comprehensive SWOT analysis.

> *Sample Study: The data reflect that 74% of the referring physicians in this market perceive a need for high-level CT studies. They are not satisfied with the hospital system now providing these services, and they do not perceive a need to have another high-field MRI source in the market. Their key service concerns are inaccessible appointment slots and lack of attention to prompt (STAT) reports from the radiology provider. Of the 74% that feel they need more comprehensive CT studies, 64% will send their patients to a new provider to get these services promptly. These group practices are heavy CT referrers. Two of the primary MRI referring sources have their own MRI scanners. No other significant barriers are identified in the research phase.*

Preparing the Research Report

The research report should include a summary of the responses to every question. The report may be in one of various reporting formats, but ultimately it is the vehicle for presenting research outcomes. The report should act as a tool by which strategic planning can begin and should bullet the elements of the SWOT analysis based on the entire assessment. It should concisely and accurately present the findings for progression into the final planning processes.

Conclusion

Research is the starting point for effective strategic decision making and planning. Being in tune with the market and customers provides direction for establishing

SIDEBAR: Developing an Effective Strategic Plan

Developing an effective strategic plan requires comprehensive data from the facility's own internal and external markets.

- Internal assessment, a two-prong process:
  - Corporate SWOT analysis.
  - Operational workflow assessment.
- External assessment:
  - Profiling the customers (patients, referring physicians, and competition).

Tackling the research process requires the organization to maintain the focus of the research objectives throughout these steps:

- Problem definition.
- Research design development (preparation).
- The research function.
- The research report.

The strategic plan wraps up the effort.

well-defined goals and objectives, a strong mission statement, and a value statement to customers that emphasizes their importance to the organization. Staff should walk away from this experience with a clear vision about their role and impact in the organization, as well as the knowledge of how to best respond to their customers.

Strategy development should not rely strictly on intuition. Solid information, in combination with intuition, helps maintain a competitive edge. Most important, good data should always be put in the hands of those individuals who will put it into action.

References

1. U.S. Department of Labor, Bureau of Labor Statistics. Occupational Outlook Handbook. Physicians and Surgeons. Available at: http://www.bls.gov/oco/ocos074.htm. Accessed May 24, 2007.

Chapter 6

What Defines Success?

Angela Colbert

Companies, departments, and employers look for an element of success when implementing protocols or designing processes. The factors for success and the measurements of success, however, are widely varied and often cause conflict and confusion. Searching for some common ground upon which to assess measurement and ultimately determine success may be a project in itself. Defining and then understanding the parameters of any project can provide some control over the achievement of success however one chooses to describe it.

For most purposes, *success* is defined as "the achievement of something desired, planned, or attempted."[1] In the realm of radiology, success can be so multifaceted that it becomes difficult to measure and even more difficult to ensure. The process of benchmarking (or looking at other companies to assess what has worked and what has not) can provide measurement tools for quality and patient care issues. However, the most difficult to measure may be the most important benchmark of all—stakeholder satisfaction and confidence.

It is helpful to note that whereas benchmarking is often used to identify and interpret industry averages, it can also be used to find best practice information. This best practice information can determine the efficacy or success of any business or clinical practice as compared with the performance of practices in similar situations (or compared to other businesses). As early as 1919, Frederick Taylor described best practice information (or benchmarking) appropriately when he noted that "among the various methods and implements used in each element of each trade there is always one method and one implement which is quicker and better than any of the rest."[2] To that end, determining success can often be as simple as improving function or predictability against a standard measure. In the case of streamlining and improving quality, the best practice benchmarking information provides that measure in the form of parameters from which one can create an objective relationship with results already obtained and assess possibilities for the future.

Where to Start?

Defining the parameters of any program is the first step to ensuring success and inspiring confidence in stakeholders. A strong set of guidelines and expected outcomes eliminates confusion throughout the process and reduces unrealistic goal setting. Further, carefully creating definable, measurable points all along the pathway promotes self-correction and enhances the ability of management to track and predict success.

For example, a multifaceted process improvement initiative must have as its final goal a variety of parameters and specific benchmarking opportunities in lieu of a broad-based increase in volume. Although increasing the volume is critical, one can best measure an overall improvement in quality and, therefore, a marketable asset if various components are decided upon and measured before, during, and after any initiative begins.

Although a plethora of information could be considered, an overall organizational quality improvement (QI) plan might include the following components:

1. Reduction in errors.
   - Fewer retakes.
   - Fewer missing or late reports.
   - Increase in regulatory compliance.

2. Increase in customer satisfaction.
   - Decrease in number of complaints.
   - Increase in overall satisfaction scoring.

3. Community involvement.
   - Increase in name recognition.
   - Increase in use of branding opportunities.
   - Increase in use of marketing and goodwill opportunities.

What to measure?

Within the defined points on the QI spectrum, one must next decide what to measure and how to measure it. For instance, a reduction in total number of radiograph retakes may signal improvement in techniques and protocol, or it may signal a decline in business overall. However, measuring retakes as a percentage of the total number of procedures will give management a feel for the success or failure of the retake portion of QI, as well as the overall increase or decrease in business. To definitively test the success of the initiative regarding retakes, one must first measure, and then assess, the current status of the facility.

If the total number of retakes in the last calendar month was 5%, this can be calculated against any present volume. Setting a benchmark of less than 2% retakes, one can measure improvement or decline against a standard. However, noting that there were 50 retakes in the preceding month and 25 in the current month may provide misleading information. Secondarily, it may be important for the facility to measure itself against competitors for best practice information and acceptable benchmark points. Therefore, it is important to look at the desired outcome against the measuring protocol.

Assessing the Baseline

One must assess where the facility is, as well as where the facility wants to be. Creating a baseline where one firmly assesses the facts promotes an environment of QI, measuring against the known. The baseline also provides information from which to actually formulate any program or improvement scenario. Additionally, assessing the situation using generic benchmarking may provide valuable best practice information to use as a guideline. Without assessing the baseline, there is no benefit to committing resources to any sort of program.

How Often Are Results Measured?

Begin with the end in mind. Many have used this phrase to describe goal setting. Creating strong end-state goals provides the organization with a framework within which to derive short- and long-term goals. Measuring too often might lead one to spend a considerable amount of time, energy, and resources on the process of measuring. Measuring too late might cause one to miss important opportunities to reassess the efficacy of the program and realign with the end-state goals.

Creating measurable short- and long-term goals that primarily affect the end-state goal can be tricky. However, it is helpful to prioritize the measurements and the system used to measure results. This prioritization should become a function of the end-state goal in relation to the baseline, along with an assessment of current facts

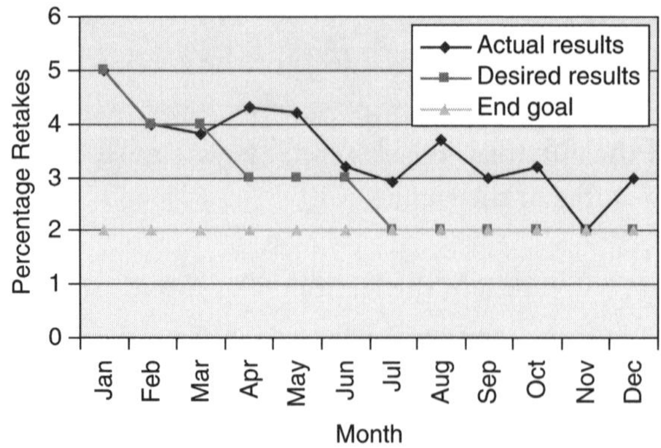

Figure 6.1 Radiograph retake improvement initiative.

and situations. For example, charting current radiograph retakes against the baseline, the end-state goal, and the short-term goal provides a visual analysis of improvement or decline (see Figure 6.1).

Using this type of visual analysis drives home the information and opens a conversation about what is working that created the results, as well as about what is not working that caused the results to deviate from the desired results and, ultimately, the end-state goal. If one were to measure the initiative monthly and assess the percentage of improvement or decline from the previous months in lieu of waiting until the end of the calendar year (as depicted in the figure), one might recognize trends, policies, procedures, or processes that support or undermine the goals. Additionally, one might create additional information points to be measured routinely to narrow down deficiencies and opportunities for growth. Additional information points might be a similar chart for each shift, each employee, or each type of study.

SIDEBAR: Tips for Defining Success

- Begin with the end in mind—a phrase that many have used to describe the process of goal setting.
- Creating an objective relationship with results may be the primary key to success in any endeavor. Doing so requires the following:
  - Establishing a baseline.
  - Setting attainable goals.
  - Measuring the progress toward the goal.

It is important to recognize, however, that the method of measuring and the data points that are being measured must be carefully weighed as to their efficacy in evoking change or providing substantive information. Again, prioritizing the measuring tools and frequency against the end goal is a reasonable step in ensuring efficiency.

Declaring Success

In Figure 6.1, the end-state goal of a consistent retake rate no greater than 2% was not achieved. However, it does appear that the facility has made substantial movement toward the goal. Celebrating even small successes, such as positive movement, may propel the rank and file toward stronger buy-in of the project and may even solicit information or ideas from the trenches. Creating ongoing opportunities for success and celebration is important to the long-term process even after the desired outcome has been reached.

Perhaps the most significant declaration of success is noting stakeholders' responses. Improved employee morale, for instance, is a strong indicator of success in any organization. Making a point of measuring all stakeholder responses may improve relations overall and be an adjunct boost to the overall process. Unexpected information may be derived from the process of communicating and noting the responses, which may prompt changes to the quality initiative.

Conclusion

Creating an objective relationship with results may be the primary key to success in any endeavor. Doing so requires (1) establishing a baseline (Where are we now?), (2) setting attainable goals (Where would we like to be?), and (3) measuring the progress toward the goal (Where is the organization in relation to where it started and where it wants to go?). Assessing the information gathered from the three steps in a logical, objective fashion creates the opportunity to course correct staff, realign vision, reallocate resources, or fine-tune goals. Using best practice benchmarking information also supports the objectivity of the process by removing emotion from the equation and providing facts to measure against. Replacing emotion with facts, and hopes with evidence, sets up the facility for the highest degree of success possible. Ultimately, however, no process can be considered truly successful without a positive impact on the stakeholders. Taking care to note subjective stakeholder satisfaction in concert with objective factual information may create the successful balance that truly propels a facility forward.

References

1. Success. *The American Heritage Dictionary of the English Language.* 4th ed. Boston, MA: Houghton Mifflin; 2004.

2. Taylor FW. *The Principles of Scientific Management.* New York, NY: Harper Bros.; 1911 :5-29.

Chapter 7

Communicating Results

Kimlyn N. Queen

> *For any radiology department to be successful, all team members within the department need to know where the department and the organization desire to go in the future. Frontline team members, all the way to the department director, need to share the same vision. The best way to ensure that all team members work toward a common goal is to create a mission and vision statement for the department that aligns with the institution's philosophy related to patient care, customer service, and commitment to the community.*

Department Mission and Vision

Once the mission and vision statements have been created, departmental goals need to be developed that will foster positive growth of the radiology department in tandem with the entire organization year after year. Developing departmental goals and clarifying mission and vision statements that will guide the actions of all team members will be effective only if all these critical elements, along with clear expectations, are properly communicated to the staff.

Without credible communication, and a lot of it, employee hearts and minds are never captured.[1] Once departmental goals have been defined, it is crucial that employees understand the goals and are willing to participate in helping the department and the institution achieve them.

For an imaging department to be successful, the departmental team members must be able to clearly define why they are there and what they want to achieve for their patients, their customers, themselves, and their organization. Developing a mission and vision statement is a way for staff to articulate these ideas to patients, customers, co-workers, administration, and the community they serve.[2]

The best way to engage employees is to include them in creating the mission and vision statements and to have them define the goals that they believe are meaningful and achievable. The following is an example of a method of gaining staff participation.

A contest was created within an imaging department as part of the mission and vision statement development process. Staff members divided into teams made up of departmental team leaders and frontline staff members. Each team created a mission statement and a vision statement. After all the teams had submitted their statements, all imaging staff members voted on the statements that they felt matched the hospital's overall mission and vision statements and truly defined their department's philosophy related to patient care, customer service, and community commitment. The winning team selected where the department director purchased lunch for the entire department the day the votes were tallied.

In this example, the mission and vision statements were as follows:

- Radiology's Mission: "To provide quality imaging services in a caring and compassionate fashion while respecting patient privacy."
- Radiology's Vision: "To provide timely service in a compassionate, caring, and friendly environment."

Vision statements may take many forms. A vision statement should answer the question, What will success look like? The purpose of a vision statement is to articulate the "dream" state of the imaging department. To help with the creation of a vision statement, one should try to answer the following questions:

1. Why do I work in this department?
2. When I move on from this department, what legacy do I want to leave behind?
3. What do I want to provide for my patients and my customers beyond the expected patient care and service?
4. If this department could be everything I dreamed, how would it be?[2]

The mission statement should describe the "what" of the department. It should explain why the department is there to provide service and what the employees are hoping to accomplish. A typical mission statement contains three components:

1. *The overall purpose of the department*—what the department and the employees are trying to achieve and why they are there.
2. *What the department does*—the types of patient care services the department provides.
3. *What is important to the employees in the department*—the values that the department will adhere to.[2]

Well-crafted mission and vision statements become the glue that binds the various parts of the imaging department together and are what drives the behaviors of the employees toward a common goal.[2]

Setting Goals and Reporting Results

Once the mission and vision statements are created, the imaging department team members should define meaningful departmental goals that the staff members want to use to demonstrate to patients and customers the department's ongoing commitment to providing quality imaging services. It is imperative that the radiology administrator or director create a format to openly and honestly communicate expectations and results on a consistent basis once the goals have been established.

The following is a sample of departmental goals that are structured in a balanced scorecard format that follows a hospital's overall goals. The balanced scorecard is broken down into four quadrants: quality, financial, customer service, and quality of work life. The goals under each quadrant are as follows:

1. Quality.
   a. Improve the departmental repeat rate from a fiscal year 2007 baseline of 3%. The goal for fiscal year 2008 is to end the fiscal year with an overall score of 3% or less.
      - Results are measured and reported by the imaging department on a monthly basis.
   b. Achieve low levels of pain (0, 1, 2, or 3 on a scale of 1 to 10) for any invasive imaging procedure for 100% of patients receiving invasive procedures. The goal for fiscal year 2008 is based on the fiscal year 2007 baseline score of 98.3%.
      - Results are measured and reported on a monthly basis by way of data collection from preprocedural and postprocedural patient surveys.
   c. Improve the accuracy of patient identification by performing the correct procedure on the correct patient (The Joint Commission patient safety standard of patient double identification). The goal for fiscal year 2008 is to have 0 radiation incidents. This goal is based on the fiscal year 2007 baseline score of 4 radiation incidents.
      - Results are measured and reported monthly based on the summary of radiation incidents for the month.

2. Financial.
   a. Meet or beat total cost per unit of service for all cost centers of responsibility. The goal for fiscal year 2008 is to be at or under budget for each imaging modality at the end of the fiscal year.
      - Results are measured and reported monthly.

b. Reduce overall expense from use of traveler technologists by $40,000. The fiscal year 2007 expense for travelers was approximately $88,000. The goal for fiscal year 2008 is to keep expenses under $48,000.

3. Customer service.
   a. Achieve a score of 81% or higher as an "overall satisfaction" score on the internal customer service report card for fiscal year 2008. This goal is based on a fiscal year 2007 baseline score of 79%.
      - Results are measured and reported monthly.
   b. Improve and achieve consistency in overall patient satisfaction for inpatients and emergency department patients. The fiscal year 2008 goal is a score of 90% or higher. The imaging department ended fiscal year 2007 with an average score of 89% for emergency department patient satisfaction and 74% for inpatient satisfaction.
      - Results are measured and reported monthly by way of Press Ganey customer satisfaction survey results.
   c. Improve the turnaround time for emergency department patient orders and procedures that exceed 45 minutes from 7:00 AM to 4:00 PM and that exceed 30 minutes from 4:00 PM to 7:00 AM. The fiscal year 2007 baseline is 98% success in overall emergency department turnaround time. The goal for the end of fiscal year 2008 is to achieve a score of 98% or 121.
      - Results are measured and reported monthly.

4. Quality of work life.
   a. Ensure a stable workforce by achieving an employee retention rate of at least 92% for fiscal year 2008. The baseline score from fiscal year 2007 was 91.75%.
      - Results are measured and reported quarterly from results calculated by the human resources department.
   b. Improve or maintain employee satisfaction survey scores to at least the hospital's overall average of 1.9. The imaging department's fiscal year 2007 baseline score was 1.6. The goal for fiscal year 2008 is to achieve a score of 1.4 or less. (The rating scale for these scores is a scale of 1 to 5, with 1 being the best score and 5 being the worst score.)
      - Results are measured and reported yearly from an employee satisfaction survey administered by the human resources department.
   c. Provide acceptable promptness and availability of studies and results for referring physicians. The goal for fiscal year 2008 is to achieve a satisfaction score of 60% or higher, with 60% representing the percentage of excellent ratings given by referring physicians on the yearly physician satisfaction survey. (Service rating selections on the survey are 1 = poor, 2 = fair, 3 = good, 4 = very good, and 5 = excellent.)
      - Results are measured and reported yearly from results of the medical staff satisfaction survey.

The radiology administrator's achievements, as well as the imaging department's performance, are based on the results of the departmental goals and how those results assist the hospital in achieving the goals set in its institutionally comprehensive balanced scorecard.

Not only is it important to consistently communicate the department's progress toward achieving goals; it is imperative that the department monitor quality assurance indicators on a monthly basis and that these quality assurance results be reported to the staff on a monthly basis.

Another important element of communicating departmental results is sharing the radiology department's progress—not just with the radiology staff but also with the radiologists, referring physicians, emergency department, nursing units, performance improvement committee, and administration. Communicate departmental results to the administration via the vice president of operations. By communicating the radiology department's results to external customers, such as the emergency department and the administration, radiology staff members are able to develop a sense of ownership and pride in producing positive results that will ultimately assist the organization as a whole in successfully achieving its goals.

Delivering the Message

There are various methods for communicating a wide variety of results. The simplest method of sharing information is monthly staff meetings that allow team members and the director to have face-to-face discussions. This strategy gives the director and the staff a chance to share successes and discuss strategies for improving results in areas that are not meeting goals. Develop a monthly schedule format of various staff meetings to ensure that all employees have an opportunity to communicate face to face with other team members and the director. A monthly meeting schedule could be structured as follows:

1. Every other month, have two imaging department meetings—at 2:00 PM and 8:00 PM—for all department employees.
2. During the months opposite the departmental meetings, the team leaders of each modality should facilitate individual staff meetings.
3. Once a month, facilitate a team leader meeting with all the modality team leaders.
4. Meet one on one each month with the team leaders.
5. Make rounds within the department twice a day with the staff to encourage informal conversations and to keep the lines of communication open at all times.

Prepare agendas, and send them out for review and input before all meetings. Take official minutes at all formal meetings, and post them for employees to read and review if they were unable to attend a meeting or if they simply want to revisit a specific topic covered during the meeting. All departmental meeting minutes should also be placed in a departmental binder for future reference and maintaining an ongoing record for The Joint Commission and any government-related inspections.

Create a monthly report, and distribute it to the vice president of operations, all radiologists, all team leaders, and the radiology RNs. The monthly report can be used as a tool to inform the recipients and staff of the department's monthly progress toward the goals defined in the departmental balanced scorecard. See Box 7.1 for an example of a monthly summary report.

Box 7.1 Sample Monthly Summary Report

Imaging Department
Monthly Report Summary
January 2006 Volumes

Month	X-ray	CT Scan	Ultrasound	CVS	Nuc Med
December	3,784	1,344	1,034	1,423	60
January	3,864	1,302	1,030	1,645	43
Y-T-D ACT	26,513	8,697	7,003	9,958	275
Y-T-D BUD	27,221	7,629	6,957	4,245	333
Prior Year for Jan. 05	3,885	1,192	1,202	1,657	46

These are monthly procedure counts. Key: Y-T-D ACT = Year to Date Actual procedure counts, Y-T-D BUD = Year to Date Budgeted procedure counts.

Quality/Service:

The month of January showed an increase in procedure counts for X-ray and CVS when compared with the month of December. The Y-T-D ACT totals for CT Scan, Ultrasound, and CVS are currently exceeding their Y-T-D BUD procedure counts.

Our quality indicators for FY-05 are:

1. Improve or maintain TAT for Emergency Department orders that exceed 45 minutes from 7 a.m. to 4 p.m. and 30 minutes from 4 p.m. to 7 a.m. from a baseline of 98% in FY-05.
2. To improve the repeat rate in X-ray from a baseline of 3% in FY-05.
3. Achieve low levels (0, 1, 2, or 3) of pain for any invasive Imaging procedure for 100% of patients receiving invasive procedures. FY-05 baseline of 98.3.
4. Improve the accuracy of performing the correct procedure on the correct patients. Measured by "radiation incidents." FY-05 baseline of 4 incidents.

For the week of January 15–21, 2006, Radiology's TAT results for ED patients were incredible, with an average score of 99.74%. This is the same level of performance that Imaging provided to the ED and ED patients in December. These ED studies were completed within acceptable time frames of 45 minutes from 7 a.m. to 4 p.m. and 30 minutes from 4 p.m. until 7 a.m. The average time for turning around an ED study dropped by 1.2 minutes to an average of 16.2 minutes per study, compared with 17.4 minutes per study during the month of December.

FY-06 ED TAT Year-to-Date Statistics

Indicator	Goal	July	Aug	Sept	Oct	Nov	Dec	Jan	Feb	March	April	May	June	FY AVG
%ED	>98%	99.21%	99.28%	98.36%	99.12%	97.78%	99.74%	99.74%						
TAT														
<30 min.														
ED Avg.	<30 Min.	17.6	16.4	19.6	18.3	18.3	17.4	16.2						
TAT														
(Min.)														

Box 7.1 (Continued)

Compared with December's score of 2.7%, our repeat rate held steady in January at an average score of 2.6%. This score is still below our departmental goal.

Our goal is to have a repeat rate of 3% or less every month. For FY-05, our average repeat rate ended at 3%. **Let's work to keep it under 3%.**

Pain Management, during Invasive Procedures, is a top priority for the Imaging Team and our patients. There were 4 procedures reported for the month of January with a 100% pain management score. Our FY-05 average, for effectiveness in controlling pain during an Invasive Procedure, was 98.3%.

There were 0 radiation incidents for the month of January. We are currently meeting our patient safety goal of performing the correct procedure on the correct patient. **GREAT JOB TEAM . . . KEEP UP THE GOOD WORK!**

Our Service Indicators for FY-05 are:

1. Achieve a minimally acceptable overall satisfaction score on the internal report card. Improve from a baseline of 79.08 in FY-05.
2. Improve and achieve consistency of customer satisfaction by reaching the 90th percentile for Press Ganey.
3. Improve inpatient customer relations by performing 3–5 patient visits per week. Results of these visits will be reflected in the Imaging Department's inpatient monthly Press Ganey Customer Service scores.

In January our Internal Report Card "Satisfaction Score" took a big leap with a score of 82.88. This is a strong increase of 2.08 compared with a score of 80.80 in December. Imaging ended FY-05 with an overall average score of 79.08. The Imaging Department works continuously with the Emergency Department and Nursing units to build and maintain positive and productive working relationships. The department administrator attends the bed meetings on a routine basis. The Imaging staff also performs weekly Nursing unit rounds. **We are confident that these actions will continue to help Imaging build stronger departmental relationships and help the hospital, as a whole, provide exceptional patient care.**

Press Ganey Percentile Rankings FY-06

Indicator	Goal	July	Aug	Sept	Oct	Nov	Dec	Jan	Feb	March	April	May	June	Average
ED Wait	90%	95%	98%	84%	92%	88%	96%	90%						
ED Courtesy	90%	87%	99%	79%	95%	96%	96%	94%						
ED Concern	90%	83%	99%	81%	96%	95%	95%	94%						
IP Wait	90%	92%	55%	91%	84%	54%	96%	87%						
IP Courtesy	90%	90%	36%	71%	79%	72%	98%	81%						

The month of January reported **GREAT** results for Imaging related to all of our ED customer service scores.

Although our inpatient customer service scores fell compared with the month of December, they still look good compared with where we were in October and November of 2005.
GREAT JOB, TEAM! KEEP UP THE AWSOME PATIENT CARE AND CUSTOMER SERVICE!
Our goal for FY-06 is to reach the 90th percentile in all categories on a consistent basis. We need to continue to work as a TEAM to increase our scores and leave our Inpatients and our ED patients with a positive and lasting impression of the exceptional care we provide them. In FY-05, we reached or exceeded the 90th percentile 30 out of 60 times, which translates into a 50% success rate. **LET'S PULL TOGETHER AND SHOW EVERYONE THAT WE ARE #1.**

LET'S STRIVE FOR THE 90'S IN FY-06.

FY-04	Average Scores	FY-05	Average Scores
ED Wait	86%	ED Wait	92%
ED Courtesy	76%	ED Courtesy	88%
ED Concern	79%	ED Concern	88%
IP Wait	69%	IP Wait	79%
IP Courtesy	66%	IP Courtesy	69%

Based on our FY-05 averages, we only met our goal of the 90th percentile in the category of ED wait times for exams; however, we showed significant improvement in all Radiology-related customer service areas. **WAY TO GO, TEAM! KEEP UP THE GREAT PATIENT CARE AND CUSTOMER SERVICE!**

JANUARY OUTCOMES FROM PATIENT VISITS

During the month of January, there were a total of 105 patient visits completed. There were 877 questions asked during these 105 patient visits, and of those 877 questions, there were 32 negative responses, or 3.6%.

Box 7.1   (Continued)

The negative responses were:

- The technologist did not introduce himself or herself (0).
- The wait was too long before being taken into the exam room (0).
- The technologist did not ask if there was anything else he or she could do for the patient before leaving the room (1).
- The patient did not receive verbal or written educational information prior to the test (16).
- Patients felt we did not demonstrate real concern for them (3).
- Patients were dissatisfied with the time frame in which their exam was performed (0).
- Patients were dissatisfied with how long it took to receive the results of their tests (0)
- Patients felt that we did not respect their privacy (0).
- Miscellaneous negative feedback (0).

For the month of January, 12 patients told us they were not given a time when they could expect their imaging procedure to be performed.

We will continue providing our patients with information about their exams and communicate procedure times to our patients and/or their families.

The breakdown of the patient visit surveys by department is as follows:

- MRI submitted 4 surveys. There were 36 questions asked of our patients. There were 4 negative responses, which gave MRI an 88.9% positive response rate.
- CT submitted 18 surveys. There were 162 questions asked of our patients. There were 6 negative responses, which gave CT a 96.3% positive response rate.
- Nuc Med submitted 7 surveys. There were 63 questions asked of our patients. There were 2 negative responses, which gave Nuc Med a 96.8% positive response rate.
- U/S submitted 23 surveys. There were 207 questions asked of our patients. There were 8 negative responses, which gave U/S a 96.1% positive response rate.
- X-ray submitted 19 surveys. There were 171 questions asked of our patients. There were 12 negative responses, which gave X-ray a 93% positive response rate.
- CVS submitted 34 surveys. There were 238 questions asked of our patients. There were 0 negative responses, for a 100% positive response rate.

Finance: Total Direct Expenses and Cost per Procedure

December	X-ray	CT Scan	Nuc Med	CVS	Ultrasound
Actual	$201,190 U	$59,928 U	$14,710 F	$17,075 F	$63,432 U
Budgeted	$200,669	$36,417	$22,684	$17,849	$41,346
Act $/Pro	$53.17 F	$44.59 U	$245.17 F	$12.00 F	$61.35 U
Bud $/Pro	$54.65	$34.19	$1031.09	$29.75	$42.58

January	X-ray	CT Scan	Nuc Med	CVS	Ultrasound
Actual	$109,295 F	$29,519 F	$20,843 F	$16,011 F	$24,113 F
Budgeted	$199,944	$36,152	$22,683	$17,364	$41,327
Act $/Pro	$28.29 F	$22.67 F	$484.72 F	$9.73 F	$23.41 F
Bud $/Pro	$51.47	$30.33	$493.11	$29.89	$34.38

This is a monthly expense chart. ACT$/PRO = Actual cost per procedure. BUD$/PRO = Budgeted cost per procedure. U = unfavorable or over budget. F = favorable or under budget.

WAY TO GO, TEAM! STAY ON A POSITIVE BUDGET COURSE!

X-ray's actual expenses came in under budget by $90,649. The Act$/Pro also came in under budget for the month of January. This is chiefly because of keeping our labor and supply expenses in line with patient volumes.

CT Scan's actual expenses and ACT$/Pro came in under budget by $6,633. This is due to a decrease in labor costs for the month of January. CT exceeded their budgeted number of procedures for January by 110 procedures.

Nuclear Medicine's actual expenses and ACT$/Pro came in under budget for the month of January. This is due to a reduction in labor costs.

Box 7.1   (Continued)

The CVS Department's actual expenses and ACT$/Pro came in under budget for the month of January. CVS exceeded their budgeted number of procedures for January by 1,064 procedures.

Ultrasound's actual expenses and ACT$/Pro came in under budget for the month of January. This came from a decrease in labor costs for the month.

There were 24 callbacks for U/S in the month of January.

There were 7 callbacks for Nuc Med in the month of January.

There were 0 callbacks for CT Scan in the month of January.

Work life/Culture

1. Ensure a stable workforce by achieving employee retention of at least 90%.
   For FY-05, our overall retention rate was 91.75%.
2. **Way to go, TEAM!** We significantly improved our 2004 employee satisfaction survey score and exceeded the hospital average of 1.7 by 0.1, for a score of 1.6 overall for Imaging. This is an improvement of 0.7 as compared with Imaging's FY-04 average score of 2.3.

The results of the Employer of Choice Survey for prior years are:

> Score for 2000 = 3.2
> Score for 2001 = 3.4
> Score for 2002 = 3.1
> Score for 2003 = 2.7
> Score for 2004 = 2.3
> Score for 2005 = 1.6

During the month of January there was a departmental pizza party to celebrate our awesome Press Ganey Scores for the month of December.

During the month of January the department had a potluck in celebration of all the January birthdays.

Next Month's Priorities:

- Continue to increase and maintain our Press Ganey scores to meet or exceed the hospital's goal of the 85th percentile.
- Focus on Retention and Improving the Employer of Choice Score.
- Continue to strengthen our patient care and customer service relationship(s) with the ED and all of our customers.
- Continue to improve our Internal Report Card results.

Prepared by Kimlyn N. Queen
Director of Imaging Service

Note that all the goals defined in the departmental balanced scorecard are reported in the monthly summary under the same format as the balanced scorecard. Doing so makes the results easy to understand and helps make the results meaningful to the radiology team members, administration, physicians, and customers.

Quality assurance indicators for the imaging department should also be divided into the four areas of the balanced scorecard:

1. Clinical quality.
    a. Misadministration of radioisotopes in nuclear medicine (goal 0).
    b. Recordable radiation-related events in nuclear medicine (goal 0).
    c. Radiation spills (goal 0).
    d. Turnaround time for all imaging reports (goal less than 8 hours).
    e. Repeat rate (goal 3% or less).
    f. Contrast complications in CT scan (goal 0).
    g. Radiation incidents in x-ray and CT scan (goal 4 or less).
    h. Unscheduled CT scanner downtime (goal 0%).
    i. Fluoro time exceeding 10 minutes (goal 0).
    j. Patient falls in imaging (goal 0).
    k. Clinical access uptime for PACS monitors (goal 98% or greater).
    l. Unscheduled downtime for all x-ray rooms (goal 0%).

2. Financial performance.
    a. Cost per procedure for all modalities (goal at or under budget).
    b. Procedure volume for all modalities (goal at or above budget).
    c. Productivity for all modalities (goal 100% or greater).

3. Customer service.
    a. Internal customer service report card score (goal 81%).
    b. Percentage of emergency department patient turnaround time within 45 minutes and 30 minutes (goal higher than 98%).
    c. Imaging customer service scores for emergency department patients (goal higher than 85%).
    d. Imaging customer service scores for inpatients (goal higher than 85%).
    e. Pain management for invasive procedures (goal 100%).

4. Quality of work life.
    a. Employee retention rate (goal 92%).
    b. Employer of choice index (goal 2.1 or lower).

Radiology administrators should create a tool for providing all imaging department quality assurance results to the CEO, all vice presidents, the peripherally inserted central venous catheter (PICC) group, and the quality assurance committee. One way to effectively communicate quality assurance results is to use a computer to download the data onto a departmental or hospital dashboard. A dashboard is a tool for progressive monitoring of departmental quality assurance performance. One can post the imaging dashboard along with quality assurance graphs every month in the department for patients, customers, and staff to view. The Sidebar shows an example of an imaging department dashboard.

SIDEBAR: Sample Dashboard

		Report Month	Benchmark	Goal	Jul	Aug	Sep	Oct	Nov	Dec	Jan	Feb	Mar	Apr	May	Jun	YTD Avg	Meeting Goal?	Calculation Warning	Ideal Direction
Marion General Hospital Dashboard FY06									Department : Imaging							Director: Kimlyn Queen				
CLINICAL QUALITY																				
CQ124	Misadministrations	Jan	0	0	0	0	0	0	0	0	0	0	0	0	0	0	0.000	TRUE	No Warning	Decrease
CQ125	Recordable Events	Jan	0	0	0	0	0	0	0	0	0	0	0	0	0	0	0.000	TRUE	No Warning	Decrease
CQ126	Radiation Spills	Jan	0	0	0	0	0	0	0	0	0	0	0	0	0	0	0.000	TRUE	No Warning	Decrease
CQ127	Turn Around Time (< 8 Hrs)	Jan	0	2.5	1.72	1.71	3.62	2.95	N/A	3.24	1.16	0	0	0	0	0	2.057	N/A	No Warning	Decrease
CQ128	Repeat Rate	Jan	0.00%	3.00%	3.50%	2.10%	2.90%	3.00%	2.00%	2.70%	2.60%	0.00%	0.00%	0.00%	0.00%	0.00%	2.69%	TRUE	No Warning	Decrease
CQ129	Complications in CT	Jan	0	0	0	0	0	0	0	0	0	0	0	0	0	0	0.000	TRUE	No Warning	Decrease
CQ130	Radiation Incidents	Jan	0	4	0	0	0	0	0	0	0	0	0	0	0	0	0.000	TRUE	No Warning	Decrease
CQ132	Unscheduled Downtime CT	Jan	0.0%	0.0%	0.0%	2.0%	5.0%	0.7%	0.0%	0.0%	0.1%	0.0%	0.0%	0.0%	0.0%	0.0%	1.1%	FALSE	No Warning	Decrease
CQ133	Fluoro exceeding 8 minutes	Jan	0	5	0	1	0	0	0	1	0	0	0	0	0	0	0.286	TRUE	No Warning	Decrease
CQ134	Fluoro exceeding 10 minutes	Jan	0	5	0	1	1	1	0	0	0	0	0	0	0	0	0.429	TRUE	No Warning	Decrease
CQ30	Patient Falls - Imaging	Jan	0	0	0	3	0	0	0	0	1	0	0	0	0	0	0.571	FALSE	No Warning	Decrease
CQ217	Clinical Access Up Time	Jan	0.0%	95.0%	100.0%	100.0%	99.0%	100.0%	100.0%	100.0%	100.0%	0.0%	0.0%	0.0%	0.0%	0.0%	99.9%	TRUE	No Warning	Increase
CQ340	Unscheduled Downtime Rad Room 1	Jan	0.0%	0.0%	1.0%	0.0%	0.1%	0.3%	0.0%	0.0%	0.0%	0.0%	0.0%	0.0%	0.0%	0.0%	0.2%	FALSE	No Warning	Decrease
CQ341	Unscheduled Downtime Rad Room 2	Jan	0.0%	0.0%	0.3%	0.0%	0.0%	0.0%	0.1%	0.0%	0.1%	0.0%	0.0%	0.0%	0.0%	0.0%	0.1%	FALSE	No Warning	Decrease
CQ342	Unscheduled Downtime Rad Room 3	Jan	0.0%	0.0%	0.0%	0.0%	0.0%	0.0%	3.0%	0.3%	0.0%	0.0%	0.0%	0.0%	0.0%	0.0%	0.5%	FALSE	No Warning	Decrease
CQ343	Unscheduled Downtime Rad Room 4	Jan	0.0%	0.0%	0.0%	0.0%	0.1%	0.0%	0.0%	0.0%	0.0%	0.0%	0.0%	0.0%	0.0%	0.0%	0.0%	FALSE	No Warning	Decrease
CUSTOMER SERVICE																				
CS300	Internal Report Card Score	Jan	0	81	81.2	81.07	79.37	79.16	82.38	80.8	62.88	0	0	0	0	0	80.980	N/A	Warning YTD Invalid	Increase
CS44	% ED Turn Around Time <30 Minutes	Jan	0.0%	98.0%	91.2%	99.3%	98.4%	99.1%	97.8%	99.7%	99.7%	0.0%	0.0%	0.0%	0.0%	0.0%	97.9%	FALSE	No Warning	Increase
CS45	ED Avg. Turn Around Time (min)	Jan	0	30	17.6	16.4	19.6	18.3	18.3	17.4	16.2	0	0	0	0	0	17.686	TRUE	No Warning	Decrease
CS46	ED Wait Time	Jan	0.0%	90.0%	95.0%	98.0%	84.0%	92.0%	88.0%	96.0%	90.0%	0.0%	0.0%	0.0%	0.0%	0.0%	91.9%	TRUE	No Warning	Increase
CS47	ED Courtesy	Jan	0.0%	90.0%	87.0%	99.0%	79.0%	95.0%	96.0%	96.0%	94.0%	0.0%	0.0%	0.0%	0.0%	0.0%	92.3%	TRUE	No Warning	Increase
CS48	ED Concern	Jan	0.0%	90.0%	83.0%	99.0%	81.0%	96.0%	95.0%	95.0%	94.0%	0.0%	0.0%	0.0%	0.0%	0.0%	91.9%	TRUE	No Warning	Increase
CS49	IP Wait Time	Jan	0.0%	90.0%	92.0%	55.0%	91.0%	84.0%	54.0%	96.0%	87.0%	0.0%	0.0%	0.0%	0.0%	0.0%	79.9%	FALSE	No Warning	Increase
CS50	IP Courtesy	Jan	0.0%	90.0%	90.0%	36.0%	71.0%	79.0%	72.0%	96.0%	81.0%	0.0%	0.0%	0.0%	0.0%	0.0%	75.3%	FALSE	No Warning	Increase
CS51	Pain Management (score <3)	Dec	0.0%	98.0%	100.0%	100.0%	100.0%	100.0%	N/A	100.0%	100.0%	0.0%	0.0%	0.0%	0.0%	0.0%	100.0%	N/A	No Warning	Increase
FINANCIAL PERFORMANCE																				
FP45	Cost per procedure X-Ray	Jan	$ -	$ 50.09	$ 52.32	$ 46.86	$ 23.27	$ 42.98	$ 39.92	$ 42.96	$ -	$ -	$ -	$ -	$ -	$ -	$ 35.47	TRUE	No Warning	Decrease
FP46	Cost per procedure MRI	Jan	$ -	$ 288.82	$ 367.45	$ 88.80	$ 247.97	$ 235.01	$ 310.81	$ 237.30	$ -	$ -	$ -	$ -	$ -	$ -	$ 212.48	TRUE	No Warning	Decrease
FP47	Cost per procedure Nuc Med	Jan	$ -	$ 477.35	$ 376.45	$ 361.76	$ 816.44	$ 275.50	$ 332.93	$ 380.78	$ -	$ -	$ -	$ -	$ -	$ -	$ 363.41	TRUE	No Warning	Decrease
FP48	Cost per procedure CT Scan	Jan	$ -	$ 32.75	$ 32.94	$ 30.52	$ 36.17	$ 47.70	$ 36.67	$ 38.58	$ -	$ -	$ -	$ -	$ -	$ -	$ 32.11	TRUE	No Warning	Decrease
FP49	Cost per procedure Ultrasound	Jan	$ -	$ 38.53	$ 26.91	$ 38.88	$ 43.41	$ 29.45	$ 46.80	$ 41.24	$ -	$ -	$ -	$ -	$ -	$ -	$ 32.38	TRUE	No Warning	Decrease
FP50	Cost per procedure CVS	Jan	$ -	$ 29.65	$ 10.18	$ 16.13	$ 10.43	$ 13.13	$ 13.35	$ 12.49	$ -	$ -	$ -	$ -	$ -	$ -	$ 10.82	TRUE	No Warning	Decrease
FP51	X-Ray Volume	Jan	0	3932	3672	3960	3943	3702	3588	3784	3864	0	0	0	0	0	3787.571	FALSE	No Warning	Increase
FP53	Nuc Med Volume	Jan	0	47	33	37	32	28	42	60	43	0	0	0	0	0	39.286	FALSE	No Warning	Increase
FP54	CT Scan Volume	Jan	0	1092	1151	1259	1246	1214	1181	1344	1302	0	0	0	0	0	1242.429	TRUE	No Warning	Increase
FP55	Ultrasound Volume	Jan	0	1033	994	1020	988	984	953	1034	1030	0	0	0	0	0	1000.429	FALSE	No Warning	Increase
FP56	CVS Volume	Jan	0	615	1474	1363	1383	1347	1323	1423	1645	0	0	0	0	0	1422.571	TRUE	No Warning	Increase
FP57	Productivity - X-Ray	Jan	0.0%	100.0%	N/A	N/A	N/A	N/A	N/A	N/A	N/A	0.0%	0.0%	0.0%	0.0%	0.0%	0.0%	N/A	No Warning	Increase
FP59	Productivity - Nuc Med	Jan	0.0%	100.0%	N/A	N/A	N/A	N/A	N/A	N/A	N/A	0.0%	0.0%	0.0%	0.0%	0.0%	0.0%	N/A	No Warning	Increase
FP60	Productivity - CT Scan	Jan	0.0%	100.0%	N/A	N/A	N/A	N/A	N/A	N/A	N/A	0.0%	0.0%	0.0%	0.0%	0.0%	0.0%	N/A	No Warning	Increase
FP61	Productivity - Ultrasound	Jan	0.0%	100.0%	N/A	N/A	N/A	N/A	N/A	N/A	N/A	0.0%	0.0%	0.0%	0.0%	0.0%	0.0%	N/A	No Warning	Increase
FP62	Productivity - CVS	Jan	0.0%	100.0%	N/A	N/A	N/A	N/A	N/A	N/A	N/A	0.0%	0.0%	0.0%	0.0%	0.0%	0.0%	N/A	No Warning	Increase
FP63	Productivity - Support	Jan	0.0%	100.0%	N/A	N/A	N/A	N/A	N/A	N/A	N/A	0.0%	0.0%	0.0%	0.0%	0.0%	0.0%	N/A	No Warning	Increase
FP52	MRI Volume	Jan	0	40	38	50	60	75	69	56	60	0	0	0	0	0	58.266	FALSE	No Warning	0
QUALITY OF WORKLIFE																				
QW21	Employee Retention Rate	Dec	0.0%	92.0%	0.0%	0.0%	99.0%	0.0%	0.0%	99.0%	0.0%	0.0%	0.0%	0.0%	0.0%	0.0%	33.0%	N/A	Warning YTD Invalid	Increase
QW60	Employer of Choice Index	Jul	0	2.1	0	0	0	0	0	0	0	0	0	0	0	0	0.000	N/A	Warning YTD Invalid	Decrease
QW600	Promptness and Availability of Studies and Results	Dec	0.0%	60.0%	0.0%	0.0%	N/A	0.0%	0.0%	N/A	0.0%	0.0%	0.0%	0.0%	0.0%	0.0%	0.0%	N/A	Warning YTD Invalid	Increase
DISCRETIONARY																				

Source: Marion (Ohio) General Hospital Imaging Department. Used with permission.

Dashboards, initially developed for business applications, are increasingly used by health systems to meet their strategic objectives. As administrators are challenged to align strategic objectives and remain competitive in the healthcare industry, they are finding that developing and implementing a dashboard with strategically balanced goals is an effective method for ensuring that each member hospital within the health system is working toward a common goal.[3]

Performance measurements have become an integral part of efforts to enhance overall performance, efficiency, and effectiveness of multiple organizations in many different industries. Dashboards are a visual representation of these measurements. Dashboards are tools that help organizations measure their performance and provide evidence to patients and customers that they are evaluating their results to determine where improvements can be made.[4] Dashboards enable organizations and employees to partner effectively to meet patient and customer needs. Dashboard metrics can include key financial indicators and measures of operational efficiencies or report on patient, customer, and employee satisfaction. Dashboard metrics should be based upon the needs of each organization and its customers. They should align the organization and staff by highlighting their interdependence in achieving service and operational excellence.[5]

In one medical group/clinical setting, for example, the data points focused on top drivers of patient satisfaction and "access satisfiers;" they were collected on a continuous basis for biweekly reporting. They included wait time for appointments, phone access, overall manner of provider, and overall quality of care.[5]

Another medical center developed a dashboard to help its group of more than a hundred physicians better focus on operational efficiency, patient satisfaction, and market growth in a managed care market. The dashboard reported a monthly snapshot of actual, target, and variance on days to third-next-available afternoon appointment, payor mix percentage, encounters per day, and length of stay.[5]

Whereas the first goal of radiology management reporting is to develop a way to document "normal" performance so that aberrations can be quickly identified and corrected, a longer-range strategic goal should be comparative reporting against the performance of other radiology groups through the use of industry benchmarks. At this time the use of industry benchmarks for creating, measuring, and reporting goals is somewhat constrained by the lack of consistent documentation of best practice information in radiology. Although benchmark information related to radiology practices is currently difficult to obtain, there are efforts in place to develop and document benchmark targets.[6]

Radiology administrators and staff members need to take high-quality imaging very seriously and report quality assurance results specific to frequently performed diagnostic radiographic procedures on a monthly basis. The philosophy behind reporting image quality assurance results is to constantly portray image quality expectations to the staff and the radiologists. Figures 7.1 and 7.2 show examples of specific diagnostic image quality assurance results. Along with specific procedural quality assurance, technologist quality assurance can be tracked for monthly numbers of examinations with proper lead marker use and technologists' initials on the images and in the PACS comment sections.

Surveying internal customers on a routine basis and communicating information and results back to them is another important aspect of creating a successful radiology department. Frontline team members should perform customer service rounds in the emergency department daily and on all nursing units weekly. The department should communicate the results of this customer service rounding in a monthly newsletter that is distributed to the emergency department, all the nursing units within the hospital, the PICC group, and the vice president of operations. See Box 7.2 for an example of a monthly newsletter communication tool.

Conclusion

Statistical data collection, information sharing, and communicating results are all critical elements of a successful radiology department. Keeping the radiology staff, administration, internal customers, external customers, and patients abreast of all the patient care processes, customer service initiatives, technologic advancements, and goals achieved within the department will help keep the department in the spotlight. However, the radiology department team members must believe in the direction that the department is moving, and the work culture has to be friendly, inviting, and nurturing.

One final, but extremely important, aspect of communication and information management in radiology that must not get lost in the data and statistical shuffle is the communication focused on recognition and celebrating individual and team achievements. If the staff members are not recognized and rewarded for their part in helping the department and the institution provide exceptional patient care and customer service, then goals will not be accomplished, morale will become negative, turnover will increase, and departmental service standards will begin to decline.

Just sharing quality assurance results, financial numbers, customer service scores, balanced scorecard (goal) results, employer-of-choice scores, retention results, and

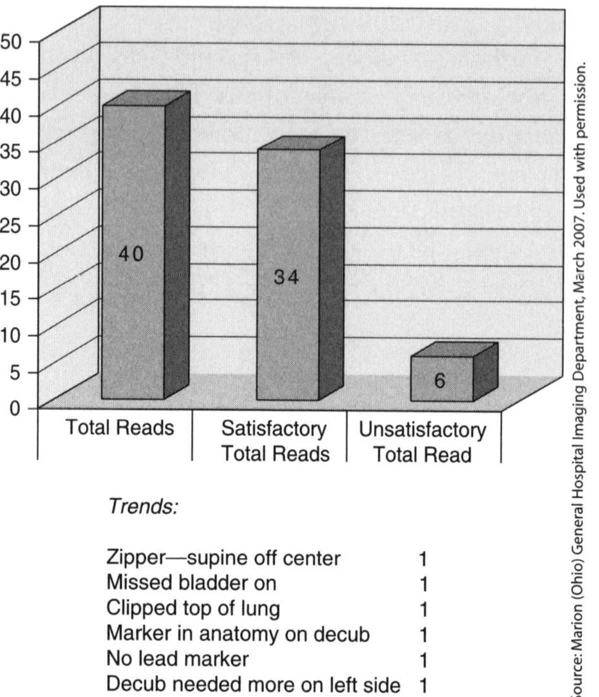

Figure 7.1 Sample quality control for acute abdominal series, December 1 through December 31.

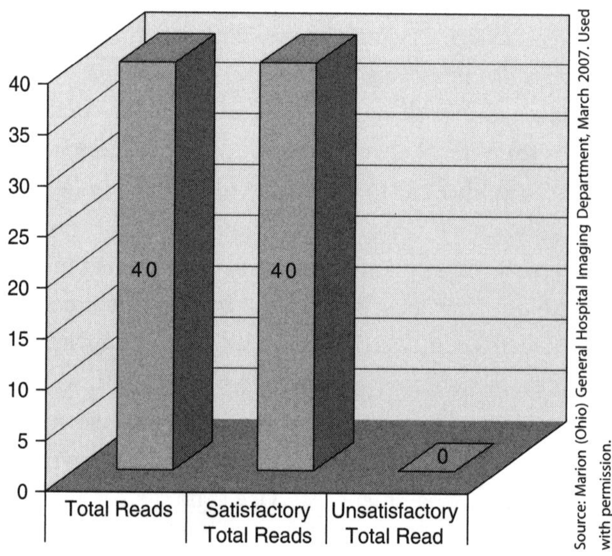

Figure 7.2 Sample quality control for portable chest radiography, December 1 through December 31.

Radiology Wants To Be Your Health Care
PARTNER . . .

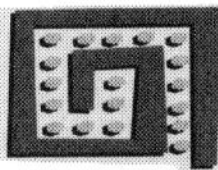

LET'S CONNECT

JANUARY, 2007, EDITION
HAPPY NEW YEAR!

What we are doing to improve our service to you and our patients:

- Daily/weekly rounds with staff on your unit
- Inpatient tests complete by 9:00 AM —December was 95.33 %
- Prior night–explanations of tests to patients
- Patient door cards to identify patients who are in Imaging and what time they went to Imaging.

Imaging's goal is to provide excellent service to all our patients. We have started by rounding with all patient care units to find out what is working and what needs to be "fixed."

Here is what we learned!

Emergency Department

Day shift made 12 "check-ins," second shift made 11, and third shift made 14, for a total of 37 "check-ins" for the month of December. Most of the comments from these "check-ins" were positive. There were a couple of reminders that were mentioned—that transporters need to remember to ask the nurse if the patient is ready for transporting, and that oxygen tanks need to be put back by the warmer in ER after a patient has been transported.

Mental Health

In December a representative of day shift made 4 visits to the Mental Health Department to see how things were going between them and the Imaging Department. She found that things were fine, and there were no complaints or problems.

ICU

In December day shift made 3 "check-ins" and second shift made 3 "check-ins" to the ICU Department. There were no problems or complaints. They said our service has been great!

1 North

There was 1 "check-in" made by second shift in December. Comments were that there were no problems and that we take good care of them.

2 North

In December day shift made 3 "check-ins," and second shift made 5 "check-ins" These rounds were all positive. There was one comment made about a clerk in the X-ray office being a great help.

2 South

In December dayshift and second shift made 5 "check-ins." All the comments were positive for the month, with no problems or concerns.

4 South

In December day shift made 5 "check-ins" with 4 South. We found that there were no problems and that everything has been fine with X-ray.

Mother/Baby

In December day shift made 2 "check-ins." We found that everything was fine, and we were told that we do a wonderful job!

Thank you for your continued feedback! We are listening! By partnering, we can make a difference with each service for our patients. Please continue to connect with us!

If you have any additional questions or comments please contact Kimlyn N. Queen, Director of Imaging, at ext. 8602, or the Administrative Secretary for Imaging at ext. 8891.

Source: Marion (Ohio) General Hospital Imaging Department. Used with permission.

physician satisfaction scores with staff members is not enough to keep them fully engaged. Thanking staff for the day-to-day work they do to help produce positive outcomes shows them that they are appreciated, that their work does make a difference, and that they are truly part of a team. Radiology is not just about technology, statistical results, and revenues; it is about patients and the people who care for them.

References

1. Kotter JP. *Leading Change*. Cambridge, MA: Harvard Business School Press; 1996.

2. Tough M. Creating a mission and vision statement. Available at: http//www.sideroad. com/Business_Communication/mission-and-vision-statement.html. Accessed April 11, 2006.

3. Developing dashboards. Original inquiry brief. Washington, DC: Marketing and Planning Leadership Council, Advisory Board Company. Available at: http:// www.advisory.com. Accessed February 21, 2003.

4. Dashboards help drive Mn/DOT performance. Available at: http://www.dot. state.mn.us/dashboards. Accessed May 15, 2006.

5. Studer Group. Give physicians real-time feedback. *Hardwire Results*. Available at: http://www.studergroup.com/newsletter/V011_Issue4/v011_i4_sec5.htm. Accessed May 9, 2006.

6. Kroken P. *Management Reporting Part I: Standard Reports and Measurements*. Reston, VA: American College of Radiology; 2004.

2 Internal and External Communications

In this section:

Chapter 8

Print Communications

Gary L. Duehring

The ability to communicate effectively in any format, including printed communications, is a key component for any successful manager. In today's healthcare environment, this skill is essential to effect efficient provision of care. Inappropriate or unclear communications not only can lead to inappropriate or endangered care but also can damage an individual's or even an organization's reputation. This chapter addresses the printed format for the transmission or communication of ideas, including memorandums, employee handbooks and manuals, newsletters, and brochures. It should be noted that printed communication also includes the production of electronically transmitted ideas and thoughts. An example would be the use of organizational e-mail for informal communications such as memorandums.

Communication, in any format, is the exchange of ideas or thoughts between two or more persons. *Effective* communication involves expressing an original message in a manner in which the recipient of the message actually receives the *intended* ideas and thoughts.

In *Management Principles for Health Professionals*, Liebler and McConnell state that communication has four components:[1]

1. *Initiation.* To initiate a communication is to enter upon or begin it. In communication, the initiation includes the cause or rationale for issuing a communication. What should the communication accomplish?
2. *Transmission.* Transmission involves sending information or a communication, or causing information to pass from one person or place to another. What form of communication is desired? This will vary with the topic or content of the printed communication.
3. *Reception.* Reception is receiving communications or information, a new idea, or a suggestion. To receive is to acquire or accept. Who is the intended recipient of the communication, and what will be the recipient's response or reaction? Who may be the nonintended recipients?
4. *Feedback.* Feedback is the process in which factors that produce a result (such as the communication of ideas or goals) are reevaluated, modified, corrected, or strengthened by the review of outcomes or results.

Communication may be initiated for a multitude of reasons, such as the following:

- To pass along a reminder.
- To provide a specific direction to the staff.
- To communicate needs or information to individuals outside the immediate department.
- To establish a policy or procedure that is needed to ensure standardization of processes or duties within the radiology department, imaging center, or group practice.

Whatever initiates the communication, the radiology administrator must ensure that it is effective.

Radiology administrators have a wide array of communication tools at their disposal. When deciding the form to use in the transmission of ideas or thoughts, either oral or printed, the radiology administrator must determine if putting the communication in print is necessary. Would a discussion be more appropriate? Is this an issue that should be addressed in a formal manner? Is a record of the discourse necessary? Is the topic of such a nature that the audience should be limited to a specific person or group?

Next, the administrator should consider how the ideas will be received by the intended audience, and possibly by a nonintended audience. Printed materials may be passed along to a far greater and varied audience than the author intended. Lastly, the administrator should expect and welcome feedback from the audience. Some feedback may be appropriate and other feedback less than appropriate, depending on the audience's reception of the communication. Is this an issue about which the administrator will invite discussion to follow, or should responses be in a printed format? Does the administrator require receipt of the communication to ensure that the intended audience was reached? Noting an avenue and timeframe for response is an excellent way to invite the audience to provide feedback.

The ability to communicate in written form is "an art and a craft."[2] Instruction in this art is outside the scope of this chapter; however, this chapter will discuss some simple rules that may help the radiology administrator effectively communicate in a professional arena.

Professionals must produce clear and concise printed communications. Radiology administrators need to produce communications meant for a recipient or audience within the organization and, occasionally, for an audience outside the organization.

When communicating it is essential to know not only the intended message but also the intended audience: "What needs to be said, and to whom?" The significant difference between oral and printed communications is that in print, the final audience may well surpass the one the author originally had in mind. The author loses control of the transmission of the communication after it is received by the intended audience. Therefore, it is important that individuals in positions of responsibility learn to produce documents that are clear, concise, accurate, and factual. They need to develop communications that are effective.

What is effective communication? Any communication, to be effective, must convey thoughts in a clear and orderly manner. The message must express the original ideas so they are understood in the same manner by the receiver as intended by the author (see Sidebar).

SIDEBAR: The 5 Cs of Communication

The following are the 5 Cs essential to clear communication:

1. *Clarity.* A message needs to be straightforward and as logically stated as possible. Very often a lack of clarity is due to an attempt to include too many ideas in the same sentence.
2. *Completeness.* Transmitting only part of a message is sometimes more harmful than no message at all.
3. *Conciseness.* Communicators must delineate the specific message they want to transfer. Most communications are enhanced when a few well-chosen words replace a verbose, carelessly worded effort.
4. *Concreteness.* Communicators usually revert to abstractions and generalizations when they are unsure about concrete facts. Choosing concrete terminology is very important.
5. *Correctness.* Flawless use of communication techniques is all in vain if the message is incorrect.

Source: Metzger N. *The Health Care Supervisor's Handbook.* 3rd ed. Salem, MA: Aspen Publishers; 1988:72-73.

Internal Communications

Internal administrative printed communications include informal writings such as memorandums (memos), reports, and simple letters. Other internal writings, such as directives, policies, and procedures, are more formal.

Memos

A *memo* is defined as "a short note written to help one remember something or remind one to do something." It is an "informal written communication, as from one

Box 8.1 Sample Staff Memo

MEMO

To: Management Staff

From: PACS Implementation Committee

Concerning: PACS update

Date: Tuesday, 6/3/07

Meeting will begin at 9:00 AM sharp. Be prepared to address proposed processes on migrating legacy data to new PACS/RIS system.

department to another in an office."[3] It has been said that a memo is a message in shirtsleeves.

The components of a memo include the author, the recipient, the subject, the date, and the body of the message. Memos should be short and specific to a topic. Remember, they are a reminder for the recipient. (See example in Box 8.1.)

The inappropriate use of memos should be avoided. Frequent, nonspecific use of memos as a convenient means of transmitting nonessential information may lead to a loss of importance for significant communications or, worse, having them ignored as "just another memo." It is helpful if all memos are posted only for a finite period and then removed.

Memos should be addressed to specific individuals for specific purposes. Radiology administrators may address memos to their management staff. Supervisors might send a memo to members of their direct line staff; however, it is inappropriate for upper management to issue memos beyond their direct line of control. This habit can diminish the authority (or perceived authority, at least) of the direct supervisor with immediate staff. Defined lines of communication need to be adhered to in both upward and downward communications. A communication from upper management intended for the entire staff should be passed along through direct supervisors.

In today's radiology departments, imaging centers, and group practices, most memos between management levels can be sent by e-mail. These electronic memos may remind individuals or groups of a meeting date and time. They may also be used to remind specific individuals of a timeline for delegated projects or to inform task groups of project progression.

Directives

A directive is a formal communication addressed to a larger audience within an organization. It can be defined as "a general instruction or order issued authoritatively."[3]

Directives should be used to define a change in practice or to redefine a point of policy. An example would be changing the dress code from laboratory coats to hospital scrubs or announcing a change in the line of command (such as announcing a new manager and his or her scope of responsibility and oversight).

Directives also are used to correct a documented procedure until a new or modified policy and procedure can be issued. An example would be altering an outdated policy on the use of gadolinium in an MRI of a lactating mother until the revised policy and procedure were published.

Directives have the expression of authority behind them and require the support of administration and all upper management. (See example in Box 8.2.)

Policy and Procedure Manuals

The most critical documentation that administrators may face is the construction and publication of a policy and procedure manual. By definition, a policy is a "principle,

---

Box 8.2 Sample Directive

DIRECTIVE

To: Imaging Personnel
Concerning: Hepatitis B vaccine

If your job description requires you to have a hepatitis B vaccine, and you feel a need for a titer or a booster, approach your supervisor for a consent form and information on scheduling these activities.

The XYZ Diagnostic Center, to provide a safe working environment, has contracted itself with Brookside Medical Center to provide services for vaccination of the center's employees who may be exposed to blood-borne hazards of hepatitis B.

Your participation will require a signed consent form (obtained from your supervisor) faxed to the Employee Health Department at Brookside Medical Center and a date and time scheduled for your visit.

Any questions should be addressed to your supervisor.

Dr. Yankess
Director, Human Resources
XYZ Diagnostic Center
6/14/07

---

plan, or course of action, as pursued by a government, organization, or individual." It represents "wise, expedient, or prudent conduct or management."[3]

Policies are written to standardize a manner of practice. Their goal is to achieve specific outcomes. Policies set the tone of the organization's culture. A well-written policy is crucial in defining the senior administration's expectation of the staff concerning certain behaviors and is an important management tool. A poorly written or nonenforced policy can be used against an organization and become a liability.

Procedures are systematic approaches that define how the staff is to ensure that a policy is met. *Webster's* states that a procedure is "the act, method, or manner of proceeding in some process or course of action; the sequences of steps to be followed."[3]

Procedures define process, whereas policies define specific expectations. Together, as a policy and procedure manual, they are the organization's self-proclaimed standards of practice to which the organization, its administration, and its staff will be held by the public, patients, referring physicians, certifying and credentialing organizations, and possibly litigating bodies. Therefore, policies and procedures should not be issued indiscriminately. They should be compiled through internal audits and participative management, and they must be strictly and consistently enforced.

Policy and procedure manuals vary from institution to institution. Some organizations may have "organizational policies," which are enforced throughout the facility, along with "departmental policies," which define the actions within a specific department such as radiology. In these cases, each body of work—both organizational and departmental—must complement the other and never be in conflict. Individuals who manage freestanding imaging centers or radiology group practices may find themselves responsible for developing everything from human resource policy and procedures to physical plant and environmental policy and procedures.

The imaging sciences and imaging departments are evolving entities. The services that these organizations offer, and how they perform them, are constantly changing. Both technology and the political environment in which healthcare operates are catalysts for change.

Examples of change caused by technologies include the introduction of computerized imaging and digital archiving. New technologies are continually being introduced (for example, PET/CT, computed radiography [CR], digital mammography, and computer-aided design [CAD] systems), and new uses of older technologies arise (for example, computed tomographic angiography [CTA] and advances in MRI technology). The political environment, through legislation such as HIPAA and mandates of the CMS, along with third-party payor directives and certification processes, also drives changes in how imaging organizations and practices operate. Therefore, policy and procedure manuals, though perpetual organizational documents, must be continually reviewed and modified to ensure appropriate outcomes. These reviews should be performed with input from each stakeholder or segment of the facility.

When developing a policy and procedure manual, it is crucial to perform an internal audit of the facility or department. This audit should answer the following questions:

- What unwritten policies and procedures are already in place that may or may not reflect the goals and intents of the organization? Who does what, and why and how do they do it?
- What issue should be addressed? Is the review of that function being done effectively?
  - Is the function being done by the right staff in the proper manner?
  - Is this function necessary?
  - Can it be performed more efficiently?
  - Does it invite an error in process that should be corrected?
  - Does it provide the outcomes that fit in the organizational goals?
- Is a new policy needed?
  - Has this issue been addressed in prior memos or directives? Is it a process or behavior that even needs to be, or should be, addressed at all?
  - Is there new legislation or regulatory mandates that need to be addressed?
  - Is there an established standard of behavior or procedure?
- If not, should there be?
  - If so, what is it, and do we meet that standard? And is it being met appropriately and universally by all concerned parties?

Policy and procedure manuals are not meant to be stored on the radiology administrator's bookshelf. Organizational or departmental policies and procedures must be distributed to all concerned parties. They must come from the highest level of authority responsible for addressing the issue, and they must be enforced by front-line management. Compliance to policies and procedures is mandatory and all-inclusive; this means that no one in any position within the organization is above compliance with these published policies and procedures.

An example of the development of a policy addressing new federal mandates on patient privacy follows:

- Operations management becomes aware of the need for new or revised policies to ensure compliance with new legislation.
- A committee of stakeholders is assembled by Operations to address the issue.
- The revisions are approved by the highest administration and legal staff.
- The policy is published by Operations.
- Frontline management ensures that all staff members are informed of, and have received, the new policy and procedure.
- The policy and procedure is enforced fairly and universally.
- Operations evaluates outcomes and validates that the organization's policy produces the required compliance with current legislation and standards. Any discovery of a need for modification must go through the same process to ensure the following:
  - Acceptance and support from senior administration.
  - Practical application in the day-to-day workflow.
  - Education of staff on how this affects them and what is expected of them.
  - Enforcement by frontline management.
  - Compliance.

Because of the changing healthcare environment, this process of review, modification, publication, implementation, and enforcement is ongoing. Organizations should have a policy and procedure in place that defines policy establishment and management. In fact, some organizations address the importance of this ongoing process by identifying an individual responsible for document control.

Policy and procedure manuals are as varied as organizations. They are specific to what an organization does and how it operates. (See example in Box 8.3.)

Employee Handbook

Imaging center and group practice administrators, along with a smaller segment of hospital radiology administrators, may be called upon to produce an employee handbook.

An employee handbook is a method of introducing newly hired personnel to the organization. It outlines general principles of employment and general public information.

Employee handbooks contain the organization's mission statement, organizational chart (lines of authority), and hours of operations. They also identify recognized

Box 8.3 Sample Policy and Procedure Manual

Injection of Contrast Media for MRI Procedures

Policy: The XYZ Diagnostic Center will use a sterile solution of the gadolinium complex for enhancement of tissue during magnetic resonance procedures as deemed appropriate by clinical examination. This injection will be performed by a registered technologist following required didactic and clinical training and proof of competency administered by a member of the center's medical staff.

Objective: To optimize the diagnostic value of MRI procedures in a safe and effective manner.

Procedure: The use of gadolinium, under the order of a physician, will be provided in accordance with FDA-approved dosages as defined in the product insert, or as specifically defined by the attending radiologist.

1. **Dosage** will be determined for:
   a. **Adults** as 0.2 mL/kg of body weight. This will be administered intravenously as a bolus injection. If required by the radiologist's directive, an additional dose may be administered at 0.4 mL/kg of body weight after a 20-minute delay after the initial injection.
   b. **Children** (2-18 years of age) as 0.2 mL/kg of body weight administered intravenously as a bolus.
   c. All injections will be followed by a flush of bacteriostatic 0.9% sodium chloride (5 mL).
2. **Indications** for the use of contrast are as follows:
   a. History of cancer or to rule out a metastatic process.
   b. To rule out an abscess or infectious process.
   c. Postoperative studies of the central nervous system.
   d. If specifically ordered by the referring physician and approved by the attending radiologist.
   e. If usage is determined medically appropriate by the attending radiologist.
3. **Limitations** to the use of contrast media follow:
   a. A medical staff member must be on the premises.
   b. Patients with a history of adverse reactions to gadolinium must have prior approval of the attending radiologist.
   c. If the patient or a responsible party refuses to give consent for contrast injection, it cannot be performed.
   d. Pregnancy is a limitation unless the procedure is ruled necessary and so documented by the referring physician and attending radiologist.

Any and all exceptions to these policies must be under the documented direction of the attending radiologist.

holidays, define pay periods, and express what the organization expects from all its employees.

Employee handbooks contain dress codes, codes of conduct, and information on in-service participation that is required of all employees regardless of their internal job classification. They define required documentation for hours worked (punching a time card, signing in, using an ID scanner, etc) and any other information new employees need to know in beginning their duties. Definitions of employee status (for example, full-time, part-time, and probationary) are also included. Employee handbooks contain the rights, privileges, and benefits the employee can expect from the organization. A general listing of the benefits is sufficient. Defining the benefits and specific processes is best handled by the human resource department or manager, as they may change over time. The handbook may also be the medium of choice to reinforce necessary general information such as parking, corporate compliance, HIPAA compliance, standards of conduct, and harassment education.

Keep this publication general. Policies and procedures do not belong in the employee handbook unless they apply to all employees. Specific job descriptions do not belong in the handbook. Any specific declarations must reflect organizational policies and not cause ambiguity.

External Communications

Professional communications outside the organization are considered formal. They should be objective in content, reflecting stated values and missions of the organization, and they should mirror organizational policies and procedures correctly and appropriately. Subjective comments should be limited and at least weighed with the question of who is going to make up the audience, remembering that these communications may reach a larger audience than intended. All printed communications to

---

SIDEBAR: Addressing Negative Customer Communications

Any customer relations communication received must be taken seriously. The radiology administrator, when faced with a customer complaint, has the opportunity to address a perceived injustice—regardless of its validity—and a thoughtful response may create strong allies from offended customers instead of alienating them and everyone else they tell of their bad experience. Complaints are the administrator's opportunity to produce good outcomes or testimonies from bad experiences. Use these opportunities to produce thoughtful responses. Remember, any response should be an effort to strengthen public relations.

In addressing any negative issue, administrators and management staff must honestly investigate and reply without admitting or assigning guilt or liability. They must be able to say, "The issue has been addressed, and we hope your next visit will be more satisfactory." It is better to discover internal problems from patient comments and resolve them than to let offended individuals disappear from the referral source or population of returning patients. Welcome the concerns of patients, and value their input. Respond in a positive manner, and attempt to foster goodwill.

external recipients should be carefully evaluated so as never to create a liability to the organization, its officers, or members of its staff (see Sidebar). Remember the 5 Cs of communication presented in the earlier Sidebar on p. 131.

Newsletters

Use any in-house publications available. The best marketing tool an organization can use is loyal word-of-mouth communications. Testimonials are repeated by patients to family members, and by employees to members of the public at large. Employees outside the radiology department need to know about the department and what services it offers. Publications with personal testimonials of positive outcomes are effective in developing public awareness and support.

Brochures

Radiology brochures that include many images and brief, specific text are easily comprehended. Collaborate with a graphics department or vendor to ensure that current information is always available to referring offices and patients. Well-formatted announcements of changes in service or operations can be faxed to referring offices. Be aware that faxes must contain information of value to the referring office or they will be perceived as a nuisance and cause future fax messages to be disregarded.

Conclusion

The nature of printed communication allows for extensive publication of information and ideas. Because the exact makeup of the audience cannot be known, it is important to prepare communications thoughtfully.

The message should be clear, complete, concise, concrete, and correct. It must be presented in proper format and be formal or informal depending on the content and intended audience. The radiology administrator must be aware of the fact that all communications represent the organization. Radiology administrators in hospital settings, imaging centers, or radiologic physician practices represent their organizations, their staff, and the radiology profession to the community they serve. The development of appropriate skills in communicating ideas is essential to succeed in administration, no matter what the field. In healthcare, outcomes are measurements of the quality of care provided. The results, or outcomes, of the transmission and reception of shared ideas, opinions, or any professional communication ultimately affect the provision of care and the staff that the administrator is responsible to lead.

References

1. Liebler J, McConnell CR. *Management Principles for Health Professionals.* 4th ed. Rockville, MD: Aspen Publishers; 2004.

2. *Publication Manual of the American Psychological Association.* 5th ed. Washington, DC: APA; 2001: 23

3. *Webster's New World Dictionary.* 4th college ed. New York, NY: Prentice Hall; 2002.

Chapter 9

Electronic Communications

Adrian Riggs

Prior to the 1990s, the typical radiology facility contained little electronic technology. A facility may have had a fax machine and perhaps a rudimentary radiology information system (RIS) interfaced with a patient database or hospital information system (HIS). Patient information was typed onto small cards for imprinting film. Internal communication was accomplished with typed documents and interoffice mail.

As technology has advanced, so has access to electronic communications. Even the most basic communication tool, the memo, has experienced a technologic upgrade because of word processing programs. Communicating imaging results has moved from delivery of films and reports to electronic transmission, and radiology staff members use state-of-the-art database programs to manage and distribute patient information.

In the imaging industry, managers communicate with department staff members, a multitude of vendors, and other departments (such as facilities, maintenance, finance, and administration). How an imaging professional communicates with others is as important as what is communicated to the intended party. The medium chosen for a communication can actually become part of the message.

Mobile Phones

In the 1990s, the best tool for contacting a radiology professional at a moment's notice was a paging device, or beeper. The caller would be at the mercy of the recipient's response time. Before the proliferation of cell phones, the recipient of a page might need to search for a pay phone or other available landline to call the paging party. Additionally, errors in the paging process or signal interruption without a verification process could cause a failure in the receipt of a page.

Today, nearly every radiology manager carries a mobile phone. The degree to which a manager is "wired" can vary dramatically; however, immediate access at any time during the workday is not only feasible but expected. With this instant access comes new responsibilities, as well as new challenges to productivity.

Business etiquette has changed in light of this technology. It is not uncommon to hear multiple phones ring during a normal business meeting. To respect the other attendees at the meeting, the radiology professional should set the mobile phone to silent (or vibrate mode, if the individual is expecting an important call).

Additionally, the cell phone user has privacy issues to consider. Because the use of the phone is no longer confined to a private office or workspace, it can be all too easy to have a conversation containing confidential subject matter in an area where others can overhear the content. Keeping the volume of the conversation low and avoiding areas with other individuals will help ensure that information is not transferred to unintended ears.

Safety is another issue with mobile phones. Many states have enacted "hands-free" laws, requiring drivers to use technology in which the phone is not held to the ear during a conversation.[1] Even with a hands-free device, a distracted driver has a higher risk of being in an accident,[2] so the user should minimize use while driving.

E-mail

E-mail has become one of the most commonly used forms of business communication. Business professionals can take the importance of e-mail for granted and do not understand the impact a single e-mail can have. Before sending an e-mail, the radiology professional should understand the importance of the e-mail's structure and content, as well as consider the audience for the message.

E-mail Etiquette

A radiology professional must recognize and observe e-mail etiquette. Just as there are informal rules when conducting business meetings, leaving phone messages, or drafting a memo, there are certain behaviors that will either enhance or detract from the intended e-mail message. More important, an e-mail message is virtually permanent. Poor etiquette practices can negatively affect the sender's perception for a long time.[3,4]

When sending e-mail messages, it is best to avoid overwhelming the reader with too much information in a format that is difficult to read. If an e-mail will contain copious amounts of information, the sender should keep the lines and paragraphs short. Bullet points or numbered items are helpful in keeping an e-mail organized and in preventing information from being lost in the message.

The grammar and punctuation used in preparing an e-mail should reflect the professional environment in which it was created. One should avoid using all capital letters, as doing so is considered shouting in an e-mail. This practice might be considered rude by the recipient and will make the message more difficult to read. Proofreading is crucial before sending an e-mail. Although an occasional typographical error will be ignored, consistent mistakes detract from the sender's professional image.[4,5]

It is important that the e-mail sender select the recipients of the e-mail message carefully. One should copy the message only to the individuals to whom it applies. Respect for others' time and e-mail inbox space is important. Abuse is demonstrated in several scenarios. For example, when an e-mail message is sent to a large group, a recipient may reply to the e-mail with a question that pertains only to one person. By replying directly to the original sender (and to only the other recipients to whom the situation applies), e-mail traffic will be kept to a minimum while still accomplishing the necessary exchange of information.[6]

When using e-mail, it is equally important to understand the possible ramifications of sending blind copies (bcc). Sending a blind copy does not guarantee that the other parties will not become aware of the practice. If the recipient of a blind copy replies to all the recipients, the other recipients can assume there was a blind copy because the address was not in the original message. This situation can lead to distrust and uncertainty and may negatively affect a professional relationship with the other parties.

Another practice that may give a recipient a negative message is the overuse of delivery/read receipts. Most e-mail programs have an option by which the sender can be notified when the recipient reads or receives the e-mail. There are instances in which this feature is appropriate, such as when it is necessary to track important document delivery. Indiscriminant use, however, can waste the recipient's time, flood the sender's inbox with receipts, and create an atmosphere of distrust.

Each e-mail message should contain an appropriate subject description. It is not uncommon for radiology managers to wade through 50 to 100 or more e-mails each day. Providing a descriptive but concise subject header improves the odds of one message standing out from others. The wording of the header may actually determine when, or if, a message is read.[7]

It is easy for e-mail to become impersonal because of its ease and speed. To avoid this, messages should begin with a greeting. The greeting should be appropriate for the relationship of the parties, such as "Hi, Mary" or "Dear Mr. Smith." Greetings should be respectful and not assume a social relationship that might offend the recipient.[8]

The closing of an e-mail is as important as the subject line and the greeting. The closing should include information that fully identifies the sender to the recipient. This information may include full name, title, company, telephone number, and other necessary contact information that will be helpful in further communications.[7,8]

Finally, the sender must carefully consider the content of the e-mail before sending it. E-mail does not show the subtleties of voice or body language. The administrator should avoid any attempts at irony or sarcasm unless certain the recipient will understand the tone. Also, a message received that causes anger should not be responded to immediately. In any case, everyone must avoid sending angry or rude messages (flaming). Sending an e-mail in anger can seriously damage a business relationship. Once an e-mail is sent, it can be impossible to retract it and avoid damage.

Creating Balance

New technology has done for e-mail what mobile phones have done for the landline telephone. Mobile e-mail devices make it possible for professionals to be in constant contact with an e-mail server. This technology is not without its disadvantages. Because more professionals are using e-mail as a standard of business communication, an individual may spend more time working e-mail than actually conducting business.

E-mail may reduce productivity if it is not controlled properly. Rarely does the sender of an e-mail expect the recipient to be poised at the computer and drop any and all tasks to reply. By making e-mail an indiscriminant priority over other tasks, the radiology professional can inadvertently set the expectation that e-mails will be answered immediately. Doing so can decrease productivity and create a situation in which expectations are never met.

SIDEBAR: E-mail Etiquette Guidelines

- Keep information concise and well organized.
- Use correct grammar and punctuation.
- Proofread!
- Select recipients carefully.
- Avoid the use of blind copies.
- Minimize "delivery/read" requests.
- Use concise subject descriptions.
- Greet the recipient appropriately.
- Close each e-mail with necessary identification information.
- Avoid flaming.

Instant Messaging (IM)

Some companies provide instant messaging (IM) programs that allow employees to have real-time conversations by computer rather than using the phone or e-mail. The advantage of this technology is speed of communication without tying up phone lines. A receptionist can IM a supervisor with a question posed by a patient who is on the phone or standing at the desk. Users can create conference IMs to distribute information quickly or entertain questions in a live, controlled forum.

Disadvantages of IM must be recognized and managed. The same technology that allows users to interact more efficiently can actually reduce productivity. Users can waste valuable time chatting with co-workers. Also, the expectation of instant response with IM can interrupt meetings or distract participants from current tasks.

Related Functionalities

E-mail is a widely used form of communication in radiology facilities, but other related program functions have also become commonplace. The use of individual and group electronic calendars, often tied to an e-mail program, has made it possible to effectively coordinate meetings and schedule conference rooms. Many mobile phones and data devices allow an administrator to synchronize the electronic calendar associated with the organization's work.

Other options include electronic folders, which provide a method by which files and data can be shared by selected users. Financial documents, departmental reports, and other large files that would normally be printed or e-mailed can reside in a folder for review by the intended recipients. Task force groups can work on a common document to ensure that version control is maintained. All these options have made it possible for most radiology managers to have a virtual secretary who coordinates, and even gives reminders of, important meetings.

Intranet

An intranet differs from the Internet in that it is a network of computers and Web sites confined to the organization's local users. Without direct or virtual access, outside users cannot participate in an intranet network. The use of an intranet environment provides connectivity and resources to intended users. The efficiency of sharing on-demand resources increases productivity by limiting the time spent on the phone with ancillary departments requesting information. An intranet also helps organize the volumes of data a radiology manager must work with during the daily activities of running a facility.[9]

As radiology facilities make the inevitable migration from film-based operations to electronic distribution of radiology images and reports, an intranet is essential for distribution of information throughout the internal part of the organization. Many electronic imaging systems allow for controlled distribution of images and reports over an intranet. The radiology manager must work closely with the information technology (IT) department to ensure that adequate representation is given for accessing the image distribution technology. Because an intranet can have Web page links similar to those on the Internet, having a link to radiology image distribution in an easy-to-find location will increase user satisfaction with the technology and decrease time spent by radiology personnel in guiding users to the correct access point.[10]

Beyond the need for image distribution, an intranet can serve many functions for the radiology manager, the radiology staff, and the entire organization. To ensure that the interests and needs of the radiology department are appropriately represented throughout the intranet, the radiology administrator must be proactive in involvement in the decision processes that determine the content and access to the intranet.[11] Input from the radiology facility on ideas for expansion of the intranet, as well as feedback on the current state of the intranet, will help provide the best resources for the facility.

An administrator should be able to utilize the organization's intranet for various tasks required when interacting with other departments. Whereas the human resources department may have the most to offer, other departments can help by interacting through the intranet. The finance department can make available commonly used forms, such as check request forms, reconciliation reports, and purchase requests.[12] This availability will ensure that managers use the most current forms and will alleviate the need for files with paper forms or duplicate desktop folders on the computer.

Besides forms, departments can communicate other useful information. The food services department can post the menu for the coming week. The compliance department can provide links to the latest training sites or certification information. The facilities department can keep users informed of upcoming disruptions in the normal flow of operations.[13] The IT department can make resources available, such as network access requests and technology guidelines.

The most commonly used resources will be from the human resources department. They may include internal job postings; the employee handbook or manual; and necessary forms for employee evaluations, position confirmation or promotion, personnel requisitions, time-off requests, and many more.

Internet

Just as an intranet facilitates communication within the "walls" of the organization, the Internet provides communication tools to individuals not connected to the internal network. Communication outside the organization ranges from operational and financial management to the marketing of department services to referring physicians, patients, and the general public. The Internet can also serve as an industry resource for other radiology facilities; the overall delivery of radiology services can be improved through the ability to access information from other radiology facilities throughout the country and beyond.[14]

Web sites are becoming the preferred method of communicating to a large audience. The hard copy Yellow Pages distributed by the local phone company may list a radiology facility's hours and modalities, but it is updated infrequently (perhaps once a year). Advertisements in the local newspaper can inform the public about upcoming health fairs or job openings; however, they are expensive and limited in content, and they can be lost in the volumes of ancillary information. A well-designed Web site, in contrast, can direct viewers to appropriate, up-to-date information.[15]

Patients

As the general use and acceptance of the Internet grows, the expectation of available information will also increase. Having a Web site that provides the radiology facility's hours and services is a good start. The Web site should also contain clinic addresses and links to maps. Specific examination preparation instructions and answers to frequently asked questions about examinations will keep the patients informed and increase the chances of successful preparation. Contact information should also be provided and should include methods by which a patient can comment about service received in the facility.

Referring Physicians

Image distribution is just as important through the Internet as it is through the organization's intranet.[10] Radiology facilities without this distribution must continue to mail and fax patient reports to referring physicians. Radiographs, when requested, must be carried by the patient or sent by mail or courier. With a properly configured electronic distribution system, the option of distributing images and reports via the organization's Web site increases the use of this technology by the referring physicians and their offices and decreases the expenses associated with a manual distribution system.

Beyond images and reports, physicians' offices have other interests that can be served by good Web site development.[3] Guidelines for ordering procedures can help minimize confusion at the time of scheduling. Scheduling itself can be facilitated with an interactive interface into the RIS.

Community

The community can also benefit from a well-designed Web site. Information on upcoming events sponsored by the radiology facility can keep the public up to date on marketing activities. Health education can be promoted as well; the Web site can give information specific to the radiology practice, as well as links to other appropriate Web sites.

Web Site Development

There are many methods by which a Web site can be developed. Although radiology facilities are relative newcomers to the Web, other businesses have studied and refined successful Web site development. Some general guidelines will help the administrator achieve the best results from the facility's Web site.[15]

The first step is to see what other facilities have done on the Web. The design team should surf the Web for content related to radiology facilities to see what is appealing and what is not. During the design process, it is important to remember that a radiology facility will be visited for specific reasons; include contact information, directions, and hours of operation. Keeping the site simple, direct, and informative will improve its success.[3,15]

Other guidelines include careful review of the content for spelling and grammar, valuable and informative links to related sites, and universal functionality. The site should work on any computer and on any browser selected. Keeping the image files small and avoiding music and sound will not only keep the site clean looking but also avoid potential incompatibilities.

Finally, most people do not encounter Web sites by accident. It is important to add promotion of the Web site into the facility's overall marketing plan. Adding the Web site URL to appointment cards and the examination report header or footer will remind customers that the site exists. The local telephone company will have Web-based directories in which the radiology site can have a direct link.

The following checklist includes pertinent criteria that should be evaluated when selecting a firm to design the radiology facility's Web site:[16]

✓ How long has the firm been designing Web sites?
✓ Does the firm have a portfolio of designs that the radiology administrator can view?
✓ What is the cost of the design, including the charge structure? What is the cost of updates throughout the life of the Web site?
✓ Who will manage and maintain the Web site?
✓ What types of training and support are available?
✓ How will the firm help the Web site attain the highest possible search engine ranking?

Conclusion

There is no doubt that technology can improve the effectiveness and productivity of the radiology administrator. Cell phones and e-mail have made it possible to communicate more efficiently. These technologies, if used properly and with the correct etiquette, can enhance the administrator's workflow and communication. Additionally, intranet and Internet use can help the radiology facility access necessary information and provide readily accessible information both internally and externally to the organization. Effective use of all these tools helps to build relationships among the staff, as well as with the facility's customers and healthcare delivery partners.

References

1. US state and local cell phone use in car legislation: Spring 2005. Available at: http://www. behandsfree.com/legislation.aspx. Accessed April 30, 2007.

2. James L. Distracted driving. Available at: http://www.drdriving.org/articles/distracted.htm. Accessed July1, 2006.

3. Goldberg G. Life online: can you email your doctor? Should you? Available at: http://www.tcs.org/ioport/dec04/emaildoc.htm. Accessed June 15, 2006.

4. Email etiquette. Available at: http://www.yourbiz.co.nz/?sectionID=63. Accessed June 23, 2006.

5. Kane B, Sands DZ. Guidelines for the clinical use of electronic mail with patients. *J Am Med Inform Assoc* 1998: 5: 104–111.

6. Bovi AM. Ethical guidelines for use of electronic mail between patients and physicians. *Am J Bioeth.* 2003; 3(3): W43–W47.

7. Ober S. *Contemporary Business Communication.* 5th ed. Boston; Houghton Mifflin Co; 2003.

8. Gaertner-Johnson L. Business writing: salutations in letters and email. Available at: http://www.businesswritingblog.com/business_writing/2006/01/greetings_ and_s.html. Accessed April 29, 2007.

9. Halamka JD. Managing care in an integrated delivery system via an intranet. In: Proceedings from the American Medical Informatics Association Annual Symposium; 1998: 401–405. Lake Buena Vista, Florida, November 7–11, 1998.

10. Brandon D. A hospital-wide distributed PACS based on intranet. *Medinfo.* 1998; 9: 1075–1079.

11. Kottmann B. Developing an intranet at Kettering Medical Center. *Intranet Journal.* Available at: http://www.intranetjournal.com/rweb/kettering-1.shtml. Accessed April 29, 2007.

12. Aymard S, Fieschi D, Volot F, Joubert M, Fieschi M. Interoperability of information sources within a hospital intranet. In: Proceedings from the American Medical Informatics Association Annual Symposium; 1998.Lake Buena Vista, Florida, November 7–11, 1998.

13. HIMSS Foundation. Web site/intranet use. Available at: http://www.himss.org/2005 survey/healthcareCIO_fina109.asp. Accessed April 29, 2007.

14. Engstrom P. Can you afford NOT to travel the Internet? *Med Econ.* 1996; 73(13): 172–4, 176, 180–1.

15. Web site guidelines for healthcare facilities—Internet. *Health Manage Technol.* April 1996. Available at: http://www.findarticles.com/p/articles/mi_m0DUD/is_n5_v17/ai_18221007. Accessed June 18, 2006.

16. Selecting a website designer. Available at: http://www.kelie.com/articles/selecting_a_ website_designer.pdf. Accessed June 21, 2006.

Chapter 10

Marketing Communications

Luis O. Marquez

Marketing communications helps businesses and organizations achieve the goals outlined in their strategic plans. It provides the mechanisms to reach key target audiences and influence their attitudes and behavior toward the facility. Among those mechanisms are direct mail, such as newsletters and brochures (see Chapter 8); networking and referral building (see Chapter 2); and advertising, public relations, and special events, all of which are discussed in this chapter.

Advertising and public relations are tools to communicate with very different audiences, have very different attributes, and achieve different goals. Because of the financial and time commitments involved, no marketing communications effort should be carried out without a detailed communications plan in place. This chapter provides basic guidance on using these valuable tools, along with special events, in support of an imaging facility's marketing efforts.

Large radiology facilities and those incorporated within hospitals or other major medical facilities often have staff responsible for marketing communications. In such cases, the radiology administrator who understands the basic principles of advertising and public relations is better able to express the radiology facility's needs to the staff members, take full advantage of their expertise, and provide effective guidance on key points to promote.

Administrators who do not have access to marketing communications or public relations professionals or staff can either hire consultants (see Box 10.1) or take on some tasks themselves. With or without professional assistance, any marketing communications efforts should begin with a communications plan.

Preparing a Communications Plan

Because there are so many ways to reach target audiences, a communications plan is an essential first step. It will focus time, attention, and funds on those tools most likely to achieve the desired goals. A plan will guide myriad decisions about which publications

---

> ### Box 10.1 Choosing and Working with a Communications Consultant
>
> Using an advertising or public relations consultant (or agency) can be a cost-effective way to achieve marketing communications goals. An experienced consultant brings knowledge and skills based on working with similar clients, best practices that an administrator is unlikely to be familiar with, an outside perspective, and credibility in the eyes of senior management. The consultant will have access to multiple vendors, such as designers and writers, and may be better able to judge their suitability for a particular project. Here are some suggestions for selecting and working with communications consultants:
>
> 1. Know what is needed. Have goals and objectives in place, or at least define the problem or issue that the consultant will address.
> 2. Match the consultant to the task. Senior consultants may have experience in both advertising and public relations, but their fees will be commensurate with that experience.
> 3. Become familiar with the types of clients the prospective consultant has worked with. The more healthcare experience the consultant has, the easier it will be to bring the consultant up to speed on the facility.
> 4. Check references, review portfolios, and understand the types of services available.
> 5. Once a consultant has been selected, create a contract that clearly outlines responsibilities, timelines, finances, and expectations.
> 6. Educate the consultant. No matter how experienced the consultant is, he or she can't know enough about the imaging facility. Provide copies of annual reports, current facility literature, organizational charts, and other basic documents to aid in planning and analysis. Put the consultant on the facility's distribution list for key documents.
> 7. Communicate with the consultant. Make sure objectives and expectations are clearly stated. Ask questions. Express concerns.
> 8. Be clear about who the contact person is, who will make the final decisions on all work produced by the consultant, and who must be included in all reviews.
> 9. Be responsive. Return calls, review submitted materials by the date agreed on (or negotiate a new date), and provide requested information in a timely fashion.
> 10. Respect the consultant, and avoid second-guessing the advice. This relationship works most effectively when both parties recognize their individual strengths and weaknesses.

to advertise in, whether to produce a brochure for a new service, and how much money to allocate in next year's budget. A well-thought-out plan will reduce costly mistakes.

A communications plan should include the following elements:

1. *Goals.* Goals are general aims that can be achieved by communications and are aligned with the organization's overall mission—for example, *to establish the imaging facility as a leader in pediatric imaging within the region.*
2. *Objectives.* Objectives are clear, concise statements of how the goals will be achieved. Objectives should include a timeframe—for example, *to create awareness of the facility's specialized pediatric services within the next 12 months.*
3. *Target audience or audiences.* When asked who needs to know, individuals creating a communications plan too often answer "everyone." Such an answer is seldom,

if ever, accurate, cost-effective, or feasible. Determining who needs to hear the message and who is most likely to act on the information provides key guidance for choosing specific communications tools. For example, possible target audiences for the goal of creating awareness of pediatric imaging services could be *pediatricians within a 20-mile radius, parents of school-aged children in the region, or editors of local children's magazines.*

4. *Key message or messages.* Communications is about sending messages, and successful marketing communications is about sending messages that accurately support the sender's mission. Key messages are used in every tool, so it is worth taking the time during the planning phase to write them out. Effective messages are simple, memorable, and relevant to the target audience. Generally, a business will identify no more than three core messages that speak to what it does and why. These messages form the basis for all communications. Specific goals may have additional key messages that reinforce the core. For example, *if a radiology facility's core message to patients emphasizes convenience, a key message for communicating about its pediatric services might be the availability of evening and weekend appointments.*

5. *Strategies and tactics.* A communications strategy defines the overall approach, and tactics are the specific tools to be used to carry out the strategy. For example, *an imaging facility whose strategy is to appeal to physicians as potential referral sources will not want to use newspaper advertising.* Table 10.1 outlines the best use of selected tactics to meet strategic needs.

6. *Budget.* The healthcare arena is a relative newcomer to the use of marketing communications, and many organizations remain reluctant to allocate sufficient funds to have an impact. This reluctance is reinforced by the difficulty in showing return on investment for some tactics. Nevertheless, it is important to outline direct and indirect costs for each tactic planned. It is wise to include costs for measuring success and, if possible, an amount for unanticipated expenses. If the total needed exceeds the funds to be allocated, the budget can help guide decisions about moving some projects into the next fiscal year or identifying alternate tactics.

7. *Implementation plan.* How will the communications be achieved, by whom, and when? These are the essential questions to be answered in this section of a communications plan. Unless someone has responsibility for a task, no one will do it. This section of the plan is particularly important for administrators who are working with public relations or marketing consultants. Projects are easily derailed if consultants and staff are duplicating efforts or consultants are stalled as they wait for staff input.

8. *Evaluation tools.* Healthcare providers are increasingly challenged to demonstrate the success or effectiveness of a procedure or medication. This demonstration is no less important in communications efforts. Successful techniques can be

Table 10.1 Comparison of Selected Marketing Communications Tactics

Tactic	Reach		Cost			Preferred Use
	Targeted	Mass	High	Medium	Low	
Newsletter	✓			✓	✓	Educate patients Attract new patients
Web site		✓	✓	✓	✓	Promotion Provide general information
E-newsletter	✓				✓	Educate patients Build relationships
Direct mail	✓			✓		Build awareness/goodwill Educate patients
Public opinion poll	✓	✓	✓	✓		Benchmarking/assessment
Advertising (print)		✓	✓	✓		Build awareness Attract new patients
Advertising (TV)		✓	✓			Build awareness Attract new patients
Advertising (radio)		✓		✓		Build awareness Attract new patients
Press release		✓			✓	Build awareness Educate community
Special events	✓		✓	✓	✓	Build goodwill Attract new patients Educate community

Source: Adapted from Hershey RC. *Communications Toolkit.* Santa Monica, CA: Cause Communications; 2005.

repeated and unsuccessful ones dropped to make way for others. Among the techniques available to measure effectiveness are the following:

- Before and after surveys or focus groups that demonstrate whether the message was received and understood.
- Response rate (for example, the number of calls for a brochure offered in an advertisement).
- Media coverage, which can range from simply counting how many times a release is used to more carefully identifying how often stories contain the key messages.
- Patient appointments, referral patterns, and other quantifiable "bottom line" data, which can be tracked according to when a specific tactic was initiated (for example, did physician referrals increase, and by how much within a specified time of advertising in a medical society publication?).

A template for a communications plan is provided in Box 10.2.

Box 10.2 Communications Plan Worksheet

Timeframe ....

Goal ....

....

Objective(s)

1. ....
2. ....
3. ....

Target Audience(s)

Objective 1
Audience(s) ....
Reason selected ....

Objective 2
Audience(s) ....
Reason selected ....

Objective 3
Audience(s) ....
Reason selected ....

Key Messages

....

....

Tactic(s)

Objective 1
Tactic .... Timeline................................

Objective 2
Tactic .... Timeline................................

Objective 3
Tactic .... Timeline................................

Budget

Tactic ....
Tactic ....
Tactic ....

Implementation Plan

Overall responsibility ....

Tactic ....
Person responsible ....
Key due dates ....

Tactic ....
Person responsible ....
Key due dates ....

Tactic ....
Person responsible ....
Key due dates ....

Measures of Success ....

....

Advertising

Advertising is paid placement of a message in a wide range of mass or targeted media. These media include newspapers, magazines, professional journals and newsletters, radio, television, Web sites and Internet search engines, nonprofit event journals (for example, a hospital auxiliary's commemorative journal), imprinted items (such as refrigerator magnets or self-examination cards), special opportunities (such as banners at events or diner placemats), and billboards.

Advertising's primary advantage is the level of control the advertiser has. If an imaging facility chooses to run a series of advertisements in local newspapers, it controls which newspapers they run in, when the advertisements run, and what messages they carry. The newspaper will send copies of the printed advertisements (called *tear sheets*) to verify publication. This provides a date from which to measure effectiveness.

Advertising can be expensive, however, so careful preplanning and assessment are essential. It can also be difficult to write and design an advertisement that will stand out from the many others, so working with a trained professional is usually warranted. The decisions of whether to advertise and in what media are influenced by four elements:[1]

1. *Reach.* This element refers to the number of people who will read, see, or hear the advertisement and is usually provided by the advertising agent. A demographic breakdown can be valuable to fully appreciate a media's reach. A daily newspaper may reach 350,000 households, but if most of these households are geographically distant from the location of a particular imaging facility, the organization will get better value for its advertising dollar if it chooses another newspaper with a more local reach.
2. *Frequency.* One of the biggest mistakes novice advertisers make is running an advertisement once or twice and then pulling it when the response does not materialize. To be effective, advertising must be repeated many times.
3. *Being memorable.* With so much competition for an audience's attention, an advertisement's message must stand out as something worth remembering. This can be accomplished with a catchy headline or slogan, an emotional appeal, or an image that the audience will immediately associate with the advertiser's message.
4. *Appropriateness.* Both the advertisement itself and the media in which it appears must be appropriate to the advertiser's goal and the target audience. An imaging facility that wants to inform physicians about new pediatric services would not use humor in its advertisement, nor would it run the advertisement on television.

Print advertising in newspapers and other media can be an effective communication tool for radiology facilities and other healthcare providers. Before an advertisement is submitted for publication, review it with the following questions in mind:[2]

- Is the message clear at a glance?
- Can the reader quickly tell what the advertisement is about?
- Does the headline include the imaging facility's major selling point?
- Does the illustration support the headline?
- Does the first line of the copy support or explain the headline and the illustration?
- Is the advertisement easy to read and understand?
- Is the type large and legible?
- Is the imaging facility clearly identified?
- Are there any excess words, phrases, or even ideas that can be deleted?
- If there is a coupon, is it easy to remove?

Public Relations

Public relations is frequently viewed as synonymous with publicity or media relations. Although it is true that publicity is an important component of most public relations efforts—and the effort on which this section focuses—public relations encompasses much more. It involves evaluating public opinion and attitudes, identifying ways to align the business or organization to the public interest, and carrying out a program that achieves public understanding.

Public relations bridges and supports the building of relationships between the healthcare organization and various publics, such as the media, local residents, employees, physicians, board members, and community leaders. Public relations creates an environment in which to accurately emphasize and build value for an existing service, a new service, or a product line. Well-executed public relations will do the following:[3]

- Increase visibility for the facility and its employees, programs, and services.
- Position the facility as a healthcare leader and authority within the community or region.
- Expand awareness of the facility's entire range of programs and services.
- Enhance the facility's image.
- Aid in recruitment and retention of employees and boost morale.
- Support efforts to raise funds for new programs and services or assist with the passage of levies and bonds.
- Act as a foundation should negative news about the facility arise.

Whereas advertising targets primarily consumers—people likely to buy the product or service promoted—public relations targets a broader group. Publics are individuals or organizations that share common interests, and they include legislators and government officials, managed care administrators, local business leaders, employees, and media reporters and editors. Public relations generally does not seek to directly influence purchasing decisions, but it can be useful to do the following:[4]

- Create and build a brand.
- Publicize the success of the business.
- Help transform a negative perception into a positive one.
- Gain a competitive advantage.
- Help launch a new or enhanced product or service.
- Help the public understand the facility's products and services.
- Announce the move into a new market.

Media Relations

The cornerstone of any publicity activity is the press release. Most readers of newspapers do not realize that many of the stories are based on, or taken entirely from, submitted press releases. These stories can be found beyond the front page and are notable because they do not carry an author's name (they do not have a by-line) (see Box 10.3).

Box 10.3 Any Imaging Facility Can Be in the News

Radiology administrators who want to build awareness through press releases to local media need only look around them for topics. Here are 15 suggestions for activities a radiology administrator could announce:

1. Changes in schedule for programs or services.
2. New staff members or partners.
3. Staff promotions.
4. Donations to local charities (services or grants).
5. New services.
6. Public seminars, workshops, or talks by physicians.
7. Special recognition, awards, or certification achieved.
8. Special business goals achieved.
9. Staff appointments to special committees or elections in professional associations.
10. New locations or reopening after renovations.
11. An open house or dedication ceremony.
12. Public events for special months (for example, National Breast Cancer Awareness month).
13. The acquisition of another practice.
14. Special screening programs.
15. Participation in health fairs or conferences.

Table 10.2 Comparison of Characteristics of Key Media Formats

Print	*Television*	*Radio*
Length of story determined by column inches or words.	Length of story can be from 15 seconds up to, but usually no more than 90 seconds.	Length of story usually 30 to 60 seconds.
Readers can reread something that doesn't make sense.	Viewers have only one opportunity to see story.	Listeners have only one opportunity to hear story.
Interviews can be done in person or over the phone.	Interviews included in story must be done in person.	Interviews can be done in person or over the phone.
Stories described through words, photographs, and graphics.	Stories described through visuals, especially action and live interviews.	Stories described through words and sounds.
Reporters cover special beats (healthcare, technology, aviation) or write for categories (business, features, sports); may also cover general assignments.	Most reporters cover general assignments or news of the day.	Reporters may have beats, but most cover general assignment.
Deadlines may be daily, weekly, or monthly depending on production schedule and number of staff reporters.	Deadlines usually day of.	Deadlines usually day or hour of.

Source: Harris and Smith Public Affairs. *Public Relations Handbook: Guidelines and Tools for Effective Public Relations.* Seattle, WA: Association of Washington Public Hospital District. Available at: http://www.awphd.org/resources_PR.asp. Accessed February 25, 2006.

The press release is a packaged article sent by a business or organization to a number of local or regional media outlets. These outlets may include newspapers, local radio and television stations, and even radiology-related magazines or journals (Table 10.2). The press release should begin with a lead paragraph containing Who, What, Where, When, Why, and sometimes How (see Box 10.4, p. 160). Although no media outlet will guarantee publication of press releases, the more polished releases will have an advantage in terms of consideration. See the Sidebar (p. 160) for some key points to keep in mind when preparing a press release.

Closely related to the press release are letters to the editor and guest editorials, or op-eds. These pieces usually contain more opinions than would a standard press release, focus on one topic of interest to a wide audience, and allow the writer to apply expertise to a community issue or support a particular point of view. They are not tools to promote a business or its services directly.

A third tool for getting publicity is the press kit, which is "a set of documents that provide the media with the foundational information they need to know about you

Box 10.4 Sample Press Release

Excellent Radiology Center
123 Smith Blvd.
Chicago, IL 60611
617-555-7890

Contact:
Don Howard, Administrator
617-555-7880

FOR IMMEDIATE RELEASE

Excellent Radiology Center Introduces Children's Exam Program

Chicago, IL, January 30, 2007–Excellent Radiology Center, which serves northwest Chicago, has introduced PediLook, a new program to reduce anxiety and stress for children who undergo nonemergency x-ray and other radiology examinations.

Developed in consultation with child life specialists and pediatricians, PediLook includes a preexamination tour for parent and child, with the option to have a doll or plush toy undergo the same procedure the child will. The day of the procedure, the child dons a special clown, princess, or cowboy costume instead of the more traditional medical gown and has a photograph taken to show friends later. Low-dose sedation is available. Parents, of course, can remain with their children at all times. A nurse makes a follow-up telephone call within 24 hours of the examination.

"A pilot program for PediLook last year produced excellent results," said Don Howard, MBA, CRA, radiology administrator for the center. "The average time needed to carry out an MRI was reduced by 10 minutes because the children were no longer reluctant to have the test. Parents were consistently pleased with the outcome and reported that their children had no signs of anxiety before or after the procedure."

Excellent Radiology Center, established in 1968, is located at 123 Smith Blvd. in the Beth-page Historical District. Its staff of seven radiologists and six registered technologists provides magnetic resonance imaging (MRI), computed tomography (CT) scans, and traditional x-ray examinations, as well as radiation therapy in association with Beth-page Medical Center and Smith Oncology Associates.

SIDEBAR: Key Points to Keep in Mind When Preparing a Press Release

- *Keep it factual.* When possible, use statistics that support the statements made in the release. Avoid hyperbole.
- *Keep it professional.* Write in the third person, and avoid slang.
- *Keep it simple.* Make the announcement. Include necessary background information, supporting data, and appropriate quotes, but keep medical terminology or jargon to a minimum. Write a brief, but strong, conclusion.
- *Keep it short.* Twelve-page press releases are not likely to be published. Try to limit the release to no more than two pages, typed and double spaced.

and your company to be able to write a story about you."[5] A press kit is analogous to an individual's curriculum vitae. The facility's best attributes and qualities need to be highlighted and packaged. Press kits are developed to generate major stories on the organization and may be prepared in support of a major event, such as the opening of a new facility.

A press kit contains multiple documents—at minimum, a press release, a fact sheet (also called a *backgrounder*) with general information about the organization or statistics related to the issue being addressed, and one or more photographs, if relevant. The information provided must be accurate, concise, relevant to the topic, and clearly presented with any medical terminology defined. Depending on the circumstances, testimonials or success stories can be included. These third-party documents are very powerful and illuminate personal interaction between the facility and the targeted audience.

None of these documents will be effective, however, if not received by the appropriate person. Keeping an accurate, up-to-date media list is an essential part of the process. Editors' and reporters' names and contact information can be found on the medium's Web site, by checking the names on healthcare or business stories that appear in the media, by looking on the print publication's masthead (often found near the editorial page in a newspaper or the table of contents in a magazine), or by calling the media outlet. Reporters and editors move frequently, so update the list at least twice a year.

Press releases can be faxed, mailed, or e-mailed. If photographs will accompany the release, digital photographs are preferred; the photograph and release should be e-mailed to the media. Press kits designed to elicit stories can be mailed to a reporter or editor; kits related to special events will usually be distributed at the event and mailed afterward to media representatives who were unable to attend.

Special Events

Staging a special event can be an effective way to reach multiple target audiences at once. For example, an open house to demonstrate a newly installed piece of equipment that introduces a significant new level of technology to the region can include physicians, the general public (potential patients), government officials, and the media. In the case of a highly technical piece of equipment, seeing is believing; a special event may be the best way to accurately communicate the message.

Nevertheless, special events can be expensive in terms of both staff time and money. Events should be incorporated into the facility's communications plan and be given the same scrutiny as other efforts before the final decision is made to proceed. No event should be planned without first defining what it is expected to accomplish. Goals might include building goodwill, educating professionals or the public, demonstrating expertise, increasing visibility with a target audience, or getting publicity. Most events achieve more than one objective, for example, garnering press attention while building goodwill.

Events are likely to succeed if they meet the needs of the target audience; fit within the facility's mission; and will be perceived as worthwhile, pleasurable, or imaginative. The following are among the types of events appropriate to an imaging facility:

- A community seminar during breast cancer awareness month.
- A facility open house or grand opening.
- A community walk-a-thon or bike-a-thon to benefit a local charity.
- An art exhibit with an opening reception featuring artwork by patients, staff, or physicians.
- A health fair, with other healthcare providers participating.
- A workshop for physicians on the latest imaging technology.
- A candlelight vigil, holiday party, or other event for cancer survivors.

Before making the final decision about holding a special event, consider the following questions:

- Is the event suitable for the community/target audience and the facility?
- Is the media likely to respond to it?
- What are its returns expected to be? What will it accomplish?
- Are the estimated costs manageable?
- Are the necessary resources available, including staff, organizational ability, and funding?
- Is everyone, from physicians to front office staff, in favor of the proposed event and prepared to support it?

A checklist for planning a special event is presented in Box 10.5.

Box 10.5 Special Events Checklist

Event .... Budget ....
Date .... Time .... Location ....
Objective ....
Coordinator...
Staff required ....
Co-sponsors ....
Target audience .... Estimated attendance ....

Publicity

	Designer	Due	Printer	Due	Distribution	Due
❑ Invitations	....	....	....	....	....	....
❑ Flyers	....	....	....	....	....	....
❑ Advertising	....	....	....	....	....	....

❑ Press release Written by... Sent ....
❑ Event photographer .... Contact info .... Confirmed ....

Speaker(s)
Name .... Contact info ....
Availability confirmed .... Bio received .... Topic reviewed ....
Accommodations: Hotel .... Airline .... Arrival ....
❑ Car/driver .... Confirmed ....
Speaker needs: ❑ Podium   ❑ Projector   ❑ Screen   ❑ Computer   ❑ VCR   ❑ DVD
❑ Other...
❑ Handouts .... Who prepares ....

Facilities/Food
❑ Rentals (chairs, etc) Items needed ....
Supplier .... Delivery to .... Time ....
....
❑ Registration
 Location .... Staffed by .... Set-up time ....
❑ Program room
 Location .... Set up by .... Set-up time ....
❑ Caterer ....Contact info .... Confirmed ....
❑ Menu ....
❑ Florist .... Confirmed ....
❑ Parking .... ❑ Valet ....

Materials

❑ Agenda	❑ Phone list with cell & after-hours numbers for key contacts
❑ Nametags	❑ Collaterals/handouts (including brochures, books to sell, etc)
❑ Sign-in sheet & pens	❑ Payment system (cash box, credit card machine)
❑ Signage to location	❑ Give-aways
❑ Signage at location	❑ Certificates/awards
❑ Seating plan/table diagram	

Supplies

❑ Pens, pencils, markers	❑ Tape	❑ Rubber bands & paper clips
❑ Extension cord & surge protector	❑ Scissors	❑ Stapler & staples

Other ....

Notes

....
....
....
....

Source: Adapted from Harris and Smith Public Affairs. *Public Relations Handbook: Guidelines and Tools for Effective Public Relations.* Seattle, WA: Association of Washington Public Hospital Districts. Available at: http://www.awphd.org/ resources_PR.asp. Accessed February 25, 2006.

Conclusion

An ongoing, well-thought-out marketing communications effort can have significant positive consequences for any business, including imaging facilities and other health-care providers. Advertising, public relations, and special events provide opportunities to inform key target audiences about available services, build credibility and goodwill, demonstrate the organization's role in the community, and influence potential patients and their referring physicians. Fortunately for busy administrators, who may not be able to call on dedicated marketing communications staff or consultants to carry out the communications plan, it can be implemented over time and still achieve its goals.

References

1. Hershey RC. *Communications Toolkit.* Santa Monica, CA: Cause Communications; 2005.

2. O'Malley J. Advertising and promotions. In: *94 Strategies for Referral Development.* San Francisco, CA: Diagnostic Imaging; 1994:71-72.

3. Harris and Smith Public Affairs. *Public Relations Handbook: Guidelines and Tools for Effective Public Relations.* Seattle, WA: Association of Washington Public Hospital Districts. Available at: http://www.awphd.org/resources_PR.asp. Accessed February 25, 2006.

4. Hasek Communications. Press kits. Available at: http://www.hasekcom.com/hasekcom/Press%20Kits.htm. Accessed February 25, 2006.

5. Crowther D. How to create press kits and online media kits. Available at: http://101publicrelations.com/presskits.html. Accessed January 2, 2006.

Chapter 11

Face-to-Face Communications

Roberta M. Edge

One of the simplest, and yet most complex, interactions in any profession is face-to-face communication—a transaction that involves sending a message, receiving it, and responding in "real time." When tone of voice, pitch, tempo, eye contact, listening skills, body language, culture, communication impairments, and differences in dialect or language are taken into account, this very basic method of communication becomes most complex. Further complexity is added when the relationships of those involved in the communications involve a hierarchy.

In this age of electronic communications, the term "face-to-face" can take on a new meaning. Synchronous communication allows people to participate at the same time regardless of time zone or physical location. Tools such as small video cameras can link people to one another by way of computer so they can "see" one another in real time yet be many miles apart. Individuals can see a presentation on the computer, dial in to a common number, hear a presenter, and watch the slides at the same time, yet never leave their offices or homes, thus sharing space electronically.[1] Asynchronous communication tools allow for communications regardless of time zone or physical space but do not permit face-to-face communications.

Albert Mehrabian is the author of a classic model regarding the feelings derived from body language in a face-to-face interaction. His research on inconsistent messages of feelings and attitudes states that 7% of meaning is derived from the words that are spoken, 38% of meaning from how we say those words and any sounds we make, and 55% of meaning from nonverbal or body language.[2] Other authors have generalized this research to spoken communication and assert that 93% of meaning in face-to-face communications is derived from sources other than the words we choose to speak (see Figure 11.1). The astute imaging administrator will relate these complexities to all types of face-to-face interactions, including discourse in staff meetings, meetings with radiologists, meetings with administration, in-house seminars, meetings with referring physicians and their office staff, focus groups, and community event sponsorship.

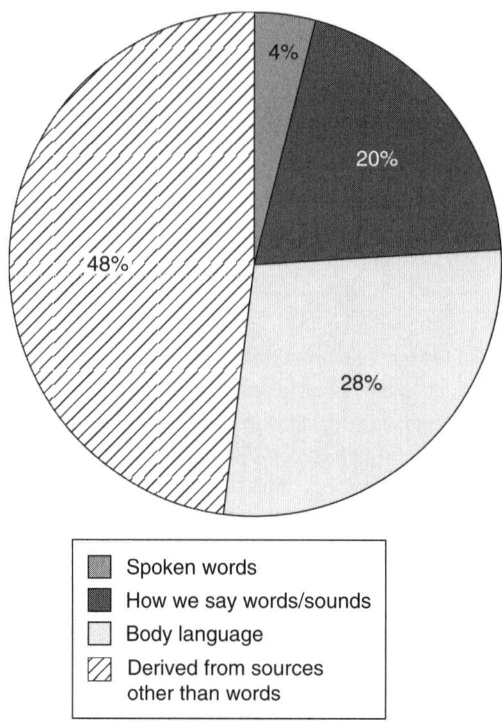

Figure 11.1 Meaning in face-to-face communication.

Components of Face-to-Face Communication

Voice (tone, pitch, and tempo), eye contact, listening skills, body language, culture, physical or mental impairments, differences in dialect or language, and hierarchy of relationships all come into play when communicating a message.

Language differences can be overcome with a good translator. The best translator is one who is physically with the patient. If such a translator is not available in the facility, a commercial service can be called upon. With all parties present, a service translator can be contacted and placed on a speakerphone to translate the messages to each party. For the patient with a hearing impairment, a translator who knows sign language can help communicate essential information. If such a translator is not available, the parties can write notes to each other. Under no circumstances should children be used to translate medical information, as their vocabulary may be limited, they may be embarrassed to translate some information, and they will not do so accurately.

Tempo of speech can be regional or cultural; for example, people in New England tend to speak more rapidly, whereas individuals in the South tend to speak more slowly. However, speaking more rapidly than normal for a particular area can be perceived as rushing to get the conversation over with, and thus mistaken as rudeness. Tone of voice and pitch can cause the listener to feel that the speaker is anything from kind to angry. Maintaining a relaxed and even tone with a midrange pitch will communicate a message clearly, without implying emotions.

Smiling while on the phone (the listener can hear the difference), keeping profanity out of any business communication, and being respectful in the delivery of face-to-face communication are all skills that can be used to enhance oral communication.[3] It is important to keep emotions, especially anger, at bay when speaking to another person in a business setting. When communication becomes heated because of anger, it is generally best to agree to revisit the issue when everyone involved has had a chance to calm themselves, and then take up the conversation from a less emotional perspective.

Body language is a term used for components of communication that include body movements or gestures that can be used with spoken words or in lieu of them.[4] Body language is driven by culture; what is perceived as pleasant in one culture may be perceived as obscene in another.

In the United States and Canada, looking at one's watch while listening to someone conveys impatience or unwillingness to really listen to the other person. Standing with arms across the chest can convey a defensive posture, whereas arms by the side can convey receptivity. Showing palms to a listener means openness; the opposite gesture of closed palms can be interpreted as hiding something. Sitting so a leg or knee points to a person means interest in that person, whereas turning away from a person means one does not want to talk to the individual.[4] A physical impairment, such as an inability to move one's arm because of a stroke, may also affect a person's body language.

When using synchronous (real-time) communication tools that do not require being able to see the other participants (such as audioconferences or webinars) or asynchronous communication tools (such as e-mail or online discussion groups), the visual cues from participating in a face-to-face encounter are lost. Therefore, miscommunication often can occur because the listener must infer meaning from the speaker using only auditory cues or only contextual cues derived from written material. When a full videoconference is used and everyone can see one another, cues from body language and the spoken word can be available and add a fuller meaning.

Assumptions also have an effect on oral communications. Several groups, including Teaching Tolerance.org (a Web project that provides free educational materials on diversity and tolerance), the Landmark Forum (a group that provides a 3-day workshop in team management and leadership), and Team Leadership (a Web site for current and past participants in the Landmark Forum), teach methods that acknowledge that we all have assumptions about our colleagues that are based on our life experiences and that we must challenge our preconceived notions to achieve understanding. Janet Lockhart and Susan Shaw, for example, describe a writing project called *re-conceiving notions*.[5] This project urges students to identify their assumptions or preconceived notions about different ethnic groups and then answer some thought-provoking questions to find out where they first came upon a particular notion, how it keeps them from seeing similarities between themselves and others, and how these assumptions might be harmful to individuals in the group.

The Landmark Forum describes *preconceived notions* as "a way of listening to people through a filter of our judgments and preconceptions which is called our 'Already Always Listening'—it is already there, and it's always there, like a running commentary of our lives."[6] Participants in seminars are asked to figure out what filter they perceive another person through, such as "she is annoying" or "he is cold and unemotional." Doing so helps the participants recognize that when they interact with an individual about whom they hold a preconceived notion, they are "already listening in a certain way," because people bring into every situation past experiences "that dictate our perceptions of everything in our present."[7] By raising their awareness of how they listen through these filters and thus listening more effectively, individuals can work to have more honest, open communications with others.

One effective communication tool is a form of listening taught in a management course based on *The 7 Habits of Highly Effective People*, by Stephen Covey. For example, in the course the facilitator describes "Habit 5: Seek First to Understand, Then to Be Understood," which is also referred to as "The Habit of Empathetic Communication." The goal is to develop the skill of "listening and responding with both the heart and mind to understand the speaker's words, intent and feelings."[8]

When listening to understand the speaker, the listener makes eye contact, focuses on the speaker, and asks questions to draw out the meaning the speaker is trying to convey. This is not the time to fix the problem; rather, the focus is on listening until the speaker's message is fully understood. Test for understanding with phrases such as the following: "I understood you to say . . . ," "So as you see it . . . ," or "As I hear it, you . . . ." Once the speaker's meaning is understood, a response to the speaker is comprehended.

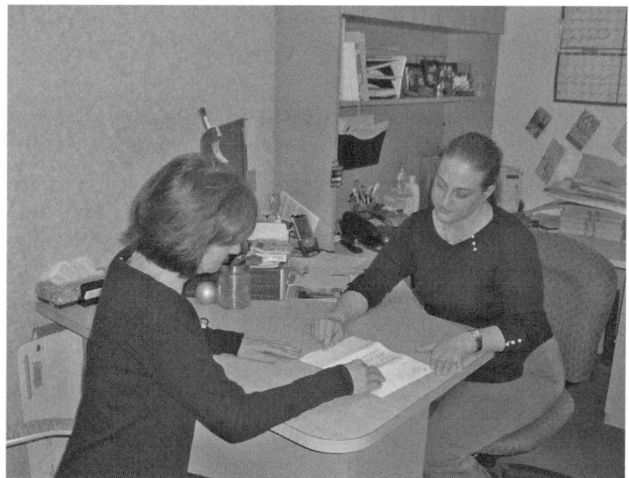

Figure 11.2 The person in the "power position" will usually sit behind a desk to convey a superior position.

The most important aspect of empathetic listening is sincerity. Empathetic listening is effective in situations in which one is not sure if one understands the message, when the speaker may not feel understood, or when an interaction is emotionally charged.[8]

We all have conversations in which we are in a superior position (in dealing with employees, for example) or an inferior position (in dealing with employers, for example). The person in the "power position" usually sits behind a desk to convey a superior position to the person spoken to (Figure 11.2). This arrangement is appropriate

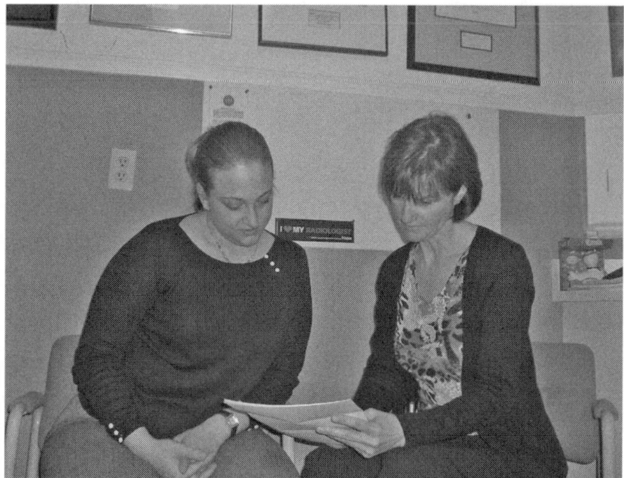

Figure 11.3 If a face-to-face encounter is one of collaboration, sitting at eye level and at arm's length is more likely to result in each person's being seen and heard.

SIDEBAR: Face-to-Face Communication Tips

1. Be mindful of voice tone, pitch, and tempo.
2. Make eye contact.
3. Listen. If the situation is emotional, listen empathetically.
4. Remember that body language communicates much of the message.
5. Take culture, dialect, and language differences into account.
6. Never use a child to translate medical information.
7. Watch out for preconceived notions that may filter messages or listening.
8. Use hierarchical positions in meetings with care.
9. Prepare an agenda for any meeting with staff members or radiologists.
10. Use the room arrangement that best facilitates communication for the type of meeting conducted.
11. Remember that radiologists and administrators are partners.
12. Remember that the administrator is the ambassador, facilitator, and model for the facility.

when hierarchy is important, such as in discussing a disciplinary issue that has gone beyond coaching or in negotiating with a vendor. If, however, the tone of the face-to-face encounter is more appropriately one of working together, then sitting at eye level and at arm's length is more likely to result in each person's being seen and heard (Figure 11.3).[9] This arrangement can be effective during an annual evaluation or coaching sessions. Equality of stature in a conversation puts both parties at ease and allows for a freer exchange of ideas.

Group Meetings

The administrator's role is generally that of facilitator. A clear voice that can be heard by all in the room is key to delivering the message, regardless of setting. With a large group a microphone may be necessary so those farthest from the speaker can hear. During a slide presentation, the speaker should continue to face the audience by placing the laptop with the presentation where it can be seen for reference. If that is not possible, the speaker should refer to note cards for each slide. Turning one's back on the audience is perceived as showing disinterest in the audience's reactions by some and as lacking professionalism by others. The projector used should present a message that is easily seen by everyone in the room.

Regardless of the type of meeting, a prepared agenda with topics and expected lengths of time for discussion helps the facilitator keep the meeting moving and allows attendees to anticipate questions and prepare input for an agenda item. An agenda keeps the meeting and participants on track; also, if there are multiple presentations, it provides a time for each presenter to arrive and make his or her presentation within the time allotted. Someone other than the facilitator should take the meeting minutes and post them for review by those not in attendance.

Room arrangement depends on the size of the audience, as well as the specific goal of the meeting. If the goal of the meeting is to brainstorm a new idea, plan workflow, team build, or begin a culture change, then small, round tables of no more than eight people per table will work best for sharing ideas.[10] Select a scribe and a spokesperson for each group. The facilitator will then collect the ideas from each table so that ideas can be collated. If the goal is to provide information, the audience is expected to follow along or to take notes. Thus, the preferred arrangement is classroom style, with rows of chairs and a center aisle, with or without a writing table in front of each row. If the group is small, everyone may be able to fit around a conference table, with the facilitator at the head of the table. Such an arrangement is appropriate for any type of meeting (see Figure 11.4).

Staff Meetings

Staff meetings are different in each organization. A staff meeting should have a facilitator and a prepared agenda, delineate a clear starting and ending time, present instructions to staff members ahead of time if they need to bring anything in particular,

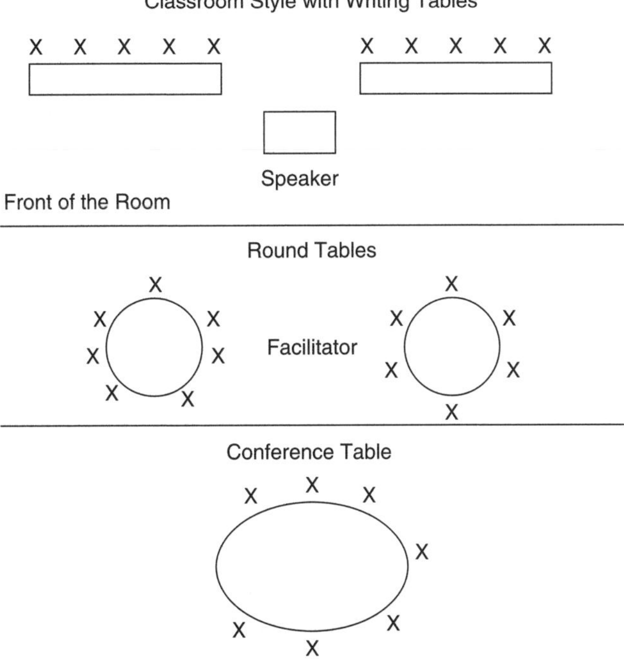

Figure 11.4 Room arrangement depends on audience size and meeting goals.

encourage participation, and include only public words of praise while avoiding negative feedback.[11] Staff meetings should be held to inform staff members of new policies and organizational goals, to train for new technology as often as needed, and to keep staff informed.[12] The meetings should be long enough to cover the materials and generally no longer than 1 hour. A 50-minute meeting may be ideal, as it causes people to be more prepared, more likely to be on time, and more focused.[13]

Radiologist Meetings

Meetings of administrators with radiologists tend to fall into one of two categories: (1) one-on-one meetings between the administrator and radiologist or (2) meetings between the entire group of radiologists and the administrator. The subject matter in these meetings revolves around three general areas: patient issues, billing, and compliance. A practice manager will participate in board meetings with a radiologist; in any other setting a radiology administrator may or may not be asked to participate in a board meeting. Remember that radiologists are partners with the administrator in the business of delivering imaging services—in the most literal sense when the administrator is running the practice, or in a figurative sense when the administrator is in a contracted setting. Keeping this in mind will help the administrator set a productive tone and emphasize working together rather than adversarial relationships.

When meeting one on one, the administrator should employ good listening skills, take notes, and get back to a particular radiologist in a timely manner when promised. The role of imaging administrator is that of ambassador when working toward a mutually beneficial outcome between the radiologist and staff. The administrator is also an advocate on issues that affect radiologists. Indeed, if there is a lack of communication between the radiologist and a staff member, the role of the administrator is to hear each side and reply to the physician and the staff member.

A common disagreement will be about the quality of images. Radiologists expect images to be of the highest quality at all times. Technologists may face challenges related to patient condition, habitus, and behavior. They may neglect to communicate the reason for suboptimal examinations, leading to frustration on the part of radiologists. If a technologist reports that a patient was in an altered state of consciousness, for example, the administrator should communicate this information to the radiologist, who will then understand and document the circumstances in the dictation of the examination. This becomes an opportunity to champion open communication between staff and radiologists. Doing so requires time and nurturing of both sides; will lead to better, more timely communication; and will build a more congenial relationship between the radiologists and staff.

In any imaging facility, the revenue stream depends on accurate billing and compliance. The administrator serves as an educator, making sure radiologists have the latest updates so their documentation is correct to maximize their billing. At times the administrator may serve as the "compliance police," ensuring that radiologists abide by the rules set by government agencies. In order to effect an appropriate change in documentation practice, meetings between the administrator and a radiologist are best held in person; alternatively, at a group meeting either the practice manager or a coding specialist might make a presentation.

At group meetings, generally the chair of the imaging department, the practice manager, or the president of the group facilitates the meeting. The administrator's job in any case is to present any operational or strategic objectives that have surfaced or need follow-up since the last meeting. The administrator may be asked to take minutes, prepare the agenda, provide a meal, or facilitate the conversation. As with other formal meetings, the agenda should be distributed before the meeting, enough time should be allotted to conduct the meeting, any audiovisual aides should be available and set up in advance of the meeting and be in working order, and the room setup should be conducive to the type of meeting. Generally, a large conference table, with the department chair or group president at the head, is most effective.

In-House Seminars

Like other professionals, radiologists and technologists are required to take continuing education courses. Some facilities offer continuing education on-site to save the cost of sending a single person off-site to a meeting; doing so spreads precious education dollars among many, if not all, staff members. This continuing education can range from bringing in a recognized speaker on a specific topic to planning a weekend-day seminar that includes 6 to 8 speakers and supplying the attendees with 6 to 8 continuing education units (CEUs), depending on the specific rules from the Recognized Continuing Education Evaluation Mechanism (RCEEM) used to approve the CEUs.

A group committed to the success of the seminar is important in planning a low-cost all-day seminar. This group ideally consists of a small number of people who will contact local physicians or technologists and get their commitment to speak.[14] Some speakers require remuneration, and some do not. Vendors may be able to help secure speakers and absorb the expense of paid speakers.

Producing a flyer or brochure announcing the seminar allows the facility to be an in-kind sponsor for the event, thus giving the facility some marketing recognition. If the facility has a marketing department, it may be willing to produce a brochure.

A facility without a marketing department can use various computer programs to create a brochure that is printed on good quality paper and is ready to be mailed. Be sure to use e-mail for recipients who prefer to be contacted electronically. If the facility has a Web site, dates and topics can be posted on it. Remember to contact nearby schools of radiologic technology, sonography, and nuclear medicine and invite their students to attend at a reduced rate.

The day of the seminar the administrator should be present to support the group and publicly acknowledge the individuals who have put on the event. Depending on budget and sponsorship, a light continental breakfast and a lunch might be served, or the attendees can be notified in advance that lunch is on their own. Advantages to including lunch are that attendees get a chance to network, they don't have to find parking again, and there won't be stragglers who may run into problems meeting the time set aside for lunch.

Be sure to provide proper audiovisual equipment, such as a microphone and laptop with projector, as most speakers will have electronic presentations. Allow time for questions, and provide handouts to the attendees so they can take notes and remember highlights from the day.

For an evening seminar, the same process applies; however the scope is smaller, the number of CEUs is lower, and a meal may or may not be offered. The advantage to offering a seminar with the evening meal is that attendees can come directly from work.

Common methods of offering CEUs include teleconferences, videoconferences, audioconferences, or webinars, all of which are synchronous (real-time) communication tools. Teleconferencing can be provided in the form of a broadcast in various locations and viewed at a specific time. Attendees sit in the same room, usually selecting a channel on a large-screen television and having a speakerphone that is muted until the audience is instructed to call in with questions. A videoconference used for classroom work involves remote attendance or distance learning. One camera is focused on the speaker, and another camera covers the audience. This allows all to "see" one another in real time and ask questions, adding to a feeling that everyone is sitting in the same room, even though separated by miles. Some larger healthcare groups use this method to hold meetings for people who all need to attend, saving some travel costs and justifying the cost saved on travel to purchase the equipment necessary to implement this type of conference. Once the equipment is paid for, there is still the cost of the connection. Videoconferences allow for in-depth discussion and feel "high touch," yet they can be costly with limited availability.[1]

Audioconferences are used to teach a course or give a presentation. They save on travel time and expenses, as each attendee dials into a common phone number and participates in his or her own office (or several people join in by speakerphone). Usually handouts of the presentation are sent out in advance and can be viewed on the attendee's computer or printed out. A newer method of audioconferencing is the webinar, a word derived from a combination of *World Wide Web* and *seminar;* the process is sometimes called *Web conferencing.* Similar to the audioconference, in a webinar there is a common dial-in number to hear the speaker, plus a Web site to log onto that is controlled by the presenter so the slides are moved at the speaker's pace. The webinar has the added feature of allowing participants to see who is online and to send questions to the speaker by way of the Web. The speaker can see the typed questions and respond to them verbally. The need for wide bandwidth and the cost can be drawbacks to these synchronous communication tools.[1]

Referring Physicians and Their Office Staff

Referring physicians are the lifeblood of an imaging facility. Without their referrals the facility would be out of business. Whether in a hospital setting, imaging center, or multispecialty physician group, maintaining a congenial relationship with refer-ring providers and their office staff is a key to success in expanding and maintain-ing the business.

Some hospitals and larger imaging facilities have a physician liaison (who may be a marketing person or a registered nurse) or a marketing person who routinely calls on referring physicians to ferret out any problems they may have in scheduling their patients in the facility. The marketing person or physician liaison is also the first line of promotion for a new service or improved piece of equipment. This liaison can bring brochures or flyers about the new equipment or service to the referring physi-cians and include a contact at the facility to speak further with them or to answer technical questions that may arise. The representative also finds out how the facility is perceived by the referring physicians and staff. Questions such as "Have you had trouble getting images or reports from us lately?" or "In the past few weeks were you able to get all your exams scheduled?" will facilitate discussion and reveal any problems.[14]

The representative should be sure to pay attention to what is going on in the waiting room of the referring physician. If it is busy with patients or other rep-resentatives are waiting, the liaison should let the staff know he or she is there and volunteer to come at another time. When representatives are able to have time with the staff or physician, they should be brief and "listen, document and follow up."[15]

If a facility does not have a marketing person or physician liaison, the job may fall to the imaging administrator to routinely contact referring physicians. With experience one learns that disgruntled referring physicians and their office staff may complain once, but they will be more likely to send their business elsewhere if they do not get a prompt reply and solution to their problems. In practice, the office staff members who schedule appointments are the key contacts. If these staff members do not get service from the imaging facility, they will, contracts permitting, send their patients to a center or hospital where their patients are taken care of in a timely manner and reports are returned to them just as promptly. By visiting the referring physicians and their staff, one develops a personal relationship and ties a face to the organization. Referring physicians are more likely to work with a facility once a relationship has been established and the facility has earned their trust.

Focus Groups

From time to time, a facility is well served by getting face-to-face feedback from customers in the form of focus groups. The composition of these groups, and the questions asked of them, should be tailored for the information the administrator wants to glean. For referral issues, physicians and their office staff are the target audience; for operational or service issues, customers who directly use the services are the target.

Generally, a third party is hired to do the interviewing and facilitate the focus group. People are usually uncomfortable giving direct face-to-face feedback, so the third-party person acts as a buffer, allowing the focus group members to be candid. A focus group can be sophisticated (for example, with the administrator and radiologists behind a two-way mirror listening in on the conversation) or simple (for example, with a marketing person facilitating the process and reporting results later).

When taking the time to gather this kind of information, it is important to demonstrate in a clear way to the participants that they have been heard and that appropriate changes have been made.

Community Events

The most likely community events in which a facility will be asked to participate are fundraisers (for the American Cancer Society or American Diabetes Association, for example), the preparation of a booth for a "disease of the month" (such as National Breast Cancer Awareness Month) or health fair, the sponsorship of a tour of the facility for a school class (such as a sixth-grade field trip to discover health careers), or team teaching a class in a business skill (such as a program in which community leaders go back to high school). No matter what the event entails, this is an opportunity for the facility to shine and garner recognition as a partner in the community where it provides imaging services.

Most fundraisers will be participatory, with the facility either sponsoring part of the event or assembling a team to raise funds for the community organization. Sponsorship may be as simple as writing a check for an advertisement in a program and underwriting the printing of a logo on a t-shirt. In contrast, sponsorship may require a physical presence, such as serving lunch or staffing the registration area. The major fundraising organizations that ask for team sponsorship are well organized and usually provide all materials necessary for the team, except a team shirt that the imaging facility provides.

Booths are fairly easy to organize; however, all protected health information (PHI) must be deleted in accordance with HIPAA. The most common booth request is for breast cancer awareness. Patients are most interested in why mammography is necessary, what the images look like, how comfortable the procedure will be, what will happen if there is an abnormal finding, and how often mammography is necessary when screening results are normal. They are also interested in ultrasonography and MRI techniques and when they are ordered. The person staffing the booth must have excellent customer service skills and be willing to engage a patient in conversation while staying within his or her scope of practice. Have brochures from the facility available with information about making an appointment. Have images that show both normal and abnormal findings (with PHI removed) and statistics that show how early cancer detection saves lives. The imaging facility may be able to provide this type of information in conjunction with the association asking for the booth, or it is readily available on the Internet to create a handout for the attendees. If a language other than English is prevalent in the area, provide handouts in both English and that language. Having a bilingual staff member who knows the subject well and is willing to attend would be an added plus for attendees who are more comfortable with their native language. The facility may also be asked to supply a raffle prize, which should be something the attendees would enjoy.

At a health fair, the facility should promote all the services it provides. Again, a variety of images, with the PHI always removed, should be displayed, along with photos of equipment. This is also an opportunity to partner with local schools of radiologic technology, sonography, and nuclear medicine to talk to people about career opportunities in imaging. Articulate staff members who are enthusiastic about their profession will add to the ambiance of the display.

Tours by local schoolchildren should be designed according to the age of the children visiting. Younger children are fascinated when able to touch or try out things on their own. When conducting those tours, one could place a child on the table to play "patient;" another child could open and close the collimators and make the table go up and down, right and left, in a regular radiographic room (with direct supervision, of course). MRI tours have many safety hazards, so it may be best to show the children the scanner from outside the room. One creative CT technologist performed a CT scan on a watermelon and gave each child a "slice" by cutting up a multiple-image film and handing one image to each child as he or she left the facility. Displays can be set up on view boxes with various images for the children to look at and ask questions about; in a PACS environment, images could be set up ahead of time on a monitor.

When visiting a school to give a guest lecture, the presenter should be prepared and allow plenty of time for questions. Most school-aged children and high school students will stay more engaged if the presentation is interactive and less of a lecture. The presenter should bring either a view box with films from different modalities or a laptop and projector to display images. The talk might include a brief anatomy lesson, an elementary discussion of the physics used to produce a radiograph, a focus on why good writing and communications skills are necessary in healthcare, a presentation of how rules used in a school (such as being on time for class) translate into any business setting, or why a career in imaging services is desirable.

Conclusion

Face-to-face communication skills are a key to success for the imaging administrator in a hospital, imaging center, multispecialty physician practice, or radiologists' practice. These communications may be one on one or in a large group. They may involve facilitating a meeting, participating in an electronic meeting, or giving a presentation.

References

1. Ashley J. Synchronous and asynchronous communication tools. *Executive Update Online.* December 2003. Available at: http://www.centeronline.org/knowledge/article.cfm?ID=2587. Accessed November 5, 2005.

2. Mehrabian A. *Silent Messages: Implicit Communication of Emotions and Attitudes.* Belmont, CA: 1981. Available at: http://www.businessballs.com/mehrabian-communications.html. Accessed November 5, 2005.

3. Lewis R. Sign up for courtesy 101. *AHRA Link.* 2002;21(1).

4. Wikipedia. Available at: http://www.en.wikipedia.org/wiki/Body_language. Accessed November 5, 2005.

5. Tolerance.org. Available at: http://www.tolerance.org/teach/web/wfc/pdf/ section_1/1_16reconceiving_notions.pdf. Accessed November 5, 2005.

6. Williams K. How my husband and I became the best of friends. Available at: http://www.teamleadership.org/landmarkforum. Accessed November 5, 2005.

7. Denison CW. *The Children of est: A Study of the Experience and Perceived Effects of Large Group Awareness Training* [PhD dissertation]. Denver, CO: University of Denver; 1994. Available at: http://www.rickross.com/reference/forum/ Art106pt3.html. Accessed May 1, 2007.

8. Covey S. *The 7 Habits of Highly Effective People.* Salt Lake City, UT: Franklin Covey; 1998.

9. Satir V. *Making Contact.* Millbrae, CA: Celestial Arts; 1976.

10. Edge R. The gift of employee dissatisfaction. *Radiol Manage.* 2002;24(1).

11. Congressional Management Foundation. Conducting staff meetings. Available at: http://www. cmfweb.org/OfficeMgmtStaffMeetings.asp. Accessed November 5, 2005

12. Huddle up—staff meetings can be fun (and useful). Available at: http://www. nfib.com/object/1583711?-templatedId=315. Accessed May 1, 2007.

13. Johnson KC. *Making* meetings more productive. *AHRA Link.* 2004;23(6).

14. Edge R. Continuing education at a reasonable cost: a case study. *Radiol Manage.* 1995;17(4).

15. Wagner P. Is silence golden? *RBMA Bull.* September/October 2003.

3 Applying Technology

In this section:

Chapter 12

Performing a Baseline Analysis

David Fox, Elisabeth Yacoback, and Patti Hoehn

The complexity of radiology administration today calls for business savvy and computerized solutions. Changes in technology during the last decade of the twentieth century, and specifically the advancements in network communications and archival media, have enabled healthcare facilities to make a transition from time-honored analog processes to what, less than 50 years ago, was mere science fiction. The fact that it is now possible to perform radiologic studies without the use of film, produce a readable interpretation of those images without the use of transcriptionist or paper, and distribute those images and reports just about anywhere to meet the needs and desires of the consumer is truly amazing. Many of these advances were merely theories only a few years ago.

For the radiology administrator, the transition to an electronic environment can be both exciting and frustrating. The costs of this technology must be managed like any other capital and operational expense, especially in light of the continuing trends of reduced reimbursement for healthcare services. Also, the costs and priorities of new technology must compete with the costs of managing existing services and planning for replacement of equipment with even newer technologies. This chapter outlines the issues associated with the development of a baseline analysis specific to information technology (IT) in the radiology environment while incorporating business principles and skills used to promote decision making for the radiology administrator.

As the radiology administrator considers either the initiation or the continuation of transition to a digital imaging environment, it is critical that a baseline analysis be conducted to identify the starting point for this transition. The baseline analysis is the foundation in planning for change. It involves documentation of the current situation as part of the strategic and tactical decision making necessary to implement any plan for the future. Simply worded, the development of a baseline analysis begins by looking at the business today, documenting the current state, and then using the current state as a benchmark for conducting a look-back. It has been said that no one starts a journey without first considering the cost, and then the journey begins with one step after another.

In this journey to a comprehensive electronic imaging environment, that first step is a series of questions:

- Where are we now with regard to IT and the management of information, both paper and electronic?
- Where do we want to go in the next 3, 5, and 10 years? (What is our vision?)
- What steps are needed to achieve these goals?
- How will changes in workflow and imaging technology affect our current systems?
- What is the condition of our current systems? What is their projected life?
- What should be addressed (for example, infrastructure, personnel, and capital)?

Baseline Assessment

Before the development of a request for proposal (RFP), before the exploration of commercial electronic information systems for the management of patient information and medical images, and even before the development of a capital strategy for technology enhancement, it is essential that a baseline assessment of the capabilities of the facility be developed. Every image management system is dependant upon a well-managed network, well-trained support staff who can troubleshoot operational issues, adequate physical space for system components, and stable power and environmental conditions. The development of a baseline assessment will evaluate these issues, along with a multitude of others, as part of the scope of the overall program.

Like any other preproject review, a SWOT analysis or similar evaluation should be conducted to identify not just needed functions or tasks but also current strengths and weaknesses of the facility, as well as opportunities for growth and even possible threats or barriers to success. In most imaging facilities, the radiology administrator is expected to have practical business acumen to employ when completing an assigned task or job. A radiology administrator who is evaluating the plausibility of implementing any type of electronic information system, however, may have to depend on expert information available within the organization, and success will be a function of the quality and quantity of that information.

A basic, step-by-step process is necessary, but it must start somewhere. For any information systems project, a good starting place is the establishment of a framework for recording information obtained from the analysis of the needs, facility, current resources, and answers to questions about future uses of the system. The radiology administrator can begin by interviewing all the potential users of the RIS or PACS.

If that community of users is too large, the radiology administrator should interview a selected subset of potential users to gather a representation of user needs.

The verbal interview process provides *subjective* (perception) information. Notes should be kept of what the potential users believe will be necessary to provide for their needs in an electronic environment, what they have heard—both positive and negative—from users of similar systems in other facilities, and what user concerns exist because of opinions formed from a literature review. The baseline analysis will progress to providing *objective* (measurable) information, which is generally obtained from the RFP in combination with analysis of the facility's strengths and weaknesses. The radiology administrator should then compare the subjective with the objective information to see if the information can improve operations and help in reaching the main goal. See Chapter 1 for more on performing baselines assessments.

The Baseline Analysis

When properly prepared and used, a baseline analysis will act as a guide for establishing a plan for the implementation of the desired information or image management system and provide a benchmark for a look-back on the value of the system in comparison with the previous methodology or operations of the facility. With this in mind, there are four recommended steps for use in formulating this analysis:

1. Establish a goal and benchmark based on historical data to see a true picture of the current state of the facility.
2. Record and organize the existing operational workflow, and determine what changes in workflow will need to occur to make the implementation of the system effective. What processes need to change, and what new processes need to be developed?
3. Diagram the current state of operational systems, paying specific attention to those systems that will need to be interfaced with the new system. What flow of information will be necessary, at what times, and at what costs?
4. Diagram the projected state of systems (where the facility wants to be), and identify the necessary steps (plan of action, strategy, and tactics) to get from the current state to the projected state. In Step 4, the costs of transition will be analyzed. Projections will be made for future costs compared with sustaining costs of the current state that will be replaced or modified.

Once carried out, these four steps can further assist the radiology administrator in identifying changes needed for a practical application involving a real-world radiology workflow issue, such as the application of IT to a traditional analog workflow.

Step 1

The first step in baseline analysis focuses on establishing a benchmark of information based on true historical data. This step allows the radiology administrator to see the current state objectively—as it is. This benchmark then provides the data to use for measuring improvement or demonstrating change. It will help a radiology administrator identify some cause-and-effect relationships and, possibly, predict the future. It is this cause-and-effect benchmark that will serve as a roadmap of an operational analysis for the implementation of any IT program. In fact, the application of any new technology must begin with an understanding of what will change or what will be affected by the changes. Every business manager or radiology administrator should know the pulse of the business at all times. These individuals must know what it is that is being measured and how the changes that are going to be implemented will affect the services provided, the people employed, and the overall cost structure of the business.

For a baseline analysis in the evaluation of an information system, several joint starting points must be addressed. Network capability and infrastructure, physical space available for IT equipment, support staff resources, training capabilities, and the availability of capital funds are only beginning points, but all will need to be addressed.

Does the facility have an adequate network infrastructure to accommodate the RIS or PACS traffic? Is it possible to separate the imaging traffic from the rest of the network traffic in the facility, or will the traffic compete for bandwidth? What is the speed or bandwidth of the network—for example, 10- or 100-Mbps? Is it fiber optic or a combination of different types of network media? How many carriers are involved? What is the network infrastructure, and is it compatible with the system being evaluated? Are the current network capabilities a strength or a weakness? In most facilities it is desirable to engage the CIO or a designated representative of this individual while answering these questions in the network analysis and roadmap development for the projected network.

In addition to an evaluation of network capabilities and needs, the baseline analysis should also identify and address physical space criteria for each component of the proposed system. What size are the servers, archive media and devices, and workstations? What type and capability of redundancy is going to be implemented, and where will the associated hardware be located? But this identification of space requirements is only a beginning. What electrical and environmental support will be needed to ensure round-the-clock services, and does the infrastructure exist to provide this support? If not, what will need to be done—and who will need to be involved—to develop and implement the necessary electrical and environmental support?

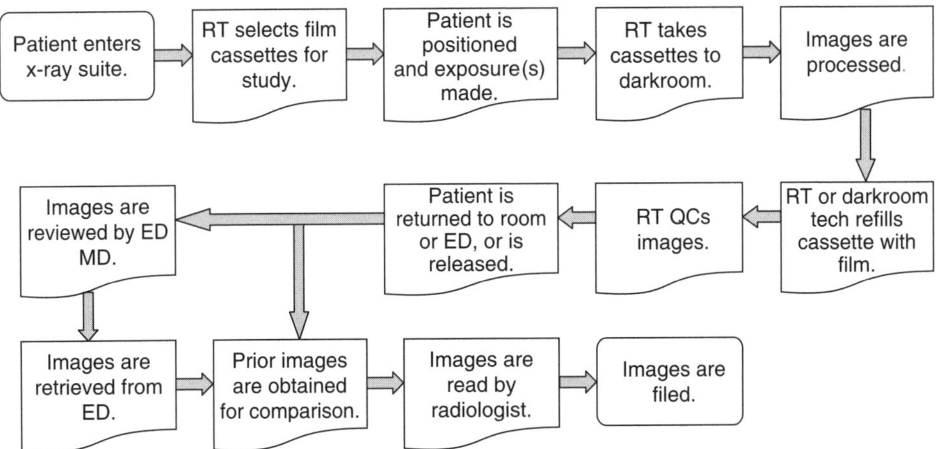

Figure 12.1 Process workflow RT indicates radiology technologist; QC, quality control; ED, emergency department; MD, doctor of medicine.

Step 2

In any analysis, the radiology administrator should remain objective. For an analysis associated with the application of new technology, and especially information or image management technology, objectivity is critical. It requires the radiology administrator to dissect current workflow and service provision procedures by taking the factual current data and recording (mapping) the findings. Mapping out the existing operational workflow in the facility that will be affected by the new technology begins with the manager—and the technology transition team, if one is being used—having a clear understanding of every process and function within the facility (Figure 12.1). This collection of data should be without strategic analysis. The strategic analysis will be conducted in Step 4.

This collection of data will need to consider each function and each workload handoff. Each and every activity, from beginning to end, should be identified so it can be evaluated for impact from the new technology (negative, positive, or no effect at all). When implementing a larger-scope project, such as the implementation of a facility-wide RIS or PACS, the workflow analysis flowcharts will be much broader in scope and detail than they would be for a smaller project, such as conversion from tape dictation to digital dictation, or a conversion from digital dictation to a speech recognition system.

At this stage of the evaluation it is best to identify personnel whose jobs will change, and especially those individuals whose jobs will no longer exist once the new technology is implemented. Retraining for workers whose job functions change can be orchestrated as part of the overall implementation plan. Developing a plan for workers whose jobs are made unnecessary because of the new technology is more difficult, but not altogether impossible. By identifying these individuals early in the evaluation process as part of the baseline analysis, new job functions or retraining to other types of jobs can be evaluated.

Step 3

Whereas Step 1 evaluated historical data and identified cause-and-effect issues within day-to-day operations, and Step 2 focused on understanding existing workflow and workflow patterns, Step 3 should focus on understanding the current operating systems, network infrastructure, and the associated power and environmental support for these systems. A diagram of the current network infrastructure should be created the same way the workflow diagram was made. The radiology administrator may need to turn to the IT department and begin to incorporate its expertise and advice into the process. Will the new technology require more bandwidth than is currently available? Will the new technology create undue stress on the current network? It is critical to understand the breaking points and effect on the institution as a whole early in the evaluation and planning process. In some situations, the use of a manual log or computer spreadsheet to document the data will assist the radiology administrator in establishing a visual snapshot of the current state (Figure 12.2).

At this stage of the evaluation it is best to identify current resources that will be available to implement and manage the new technology. What personnel are available to assume responsibility for initial and ongoing training? What personnel will manage the technology? Will it be a single individual or a group of individuals with different skill sets (for example, technicians, engineers, and programmers)? Together these tasks will give the radiology administrator an understanding of the

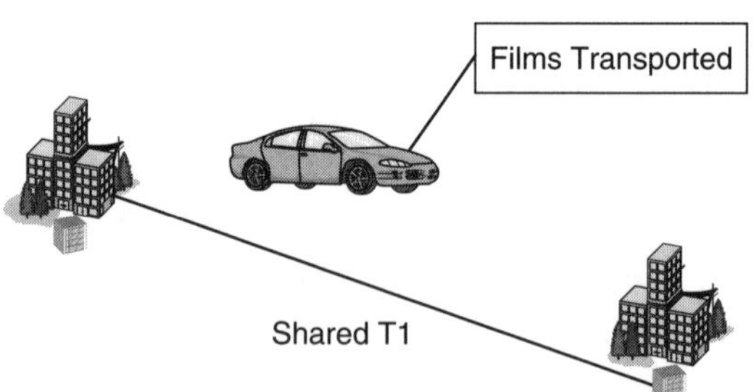

Figure 12.2 Visual snapshot for the current state of operations Hospital XYZ has a satellite screening mammography office in a shopping mall 20 miles from the hospital itself. The radiology administrator is exploring conversion to digital mammography and has mapped out the process flow and network infrastructure of the current state of operations. Mammography studies are obtained on film, with patient and examination demographics transmitted by way of a T1 telephone line. Radiographs are transported by car for reading at the end of the day.

dependency relationships between current workflow and current operating systems, as well as of what cause-and-effect relationships will need to be identified, addressed, and reviewed as part of the new technology implementation.

Step 4

Step 4 of the analysis is the most complex and time-consuming. In this step, the radiology administrator, project team, or both will diagram the projected state of systems (the desired goal) and conclude by identifying the steps (plan of action, strategy, and tactics) necessary to get from the current state to the projected state. Included in Step 4 is an exploration of increases in operational costs and any necessary capital costs that will be incurred by the project.

After workflow and operational systems analyses and flowcharts have been made, the next step in the development of a baseline analysis for technology changes is to update the previous work with the new functions or new processes obtained from the changes in technology. A new process workflow will be developed to outline the new process and show how the new technology adds or deletes steps in the existing process (Figure 12.3).

Once a reasonable assessment of process and systems changes has been completed, it is necessary to identify any increases in operating costs that will be generated by the change in technology, as well as any capital monies that will be necessary for the acquisition and implementation of the project. As part of a comprehensive baseline analysis, the radiology administrator should generate at least a basic financial statement that identifies return on investment for the project.

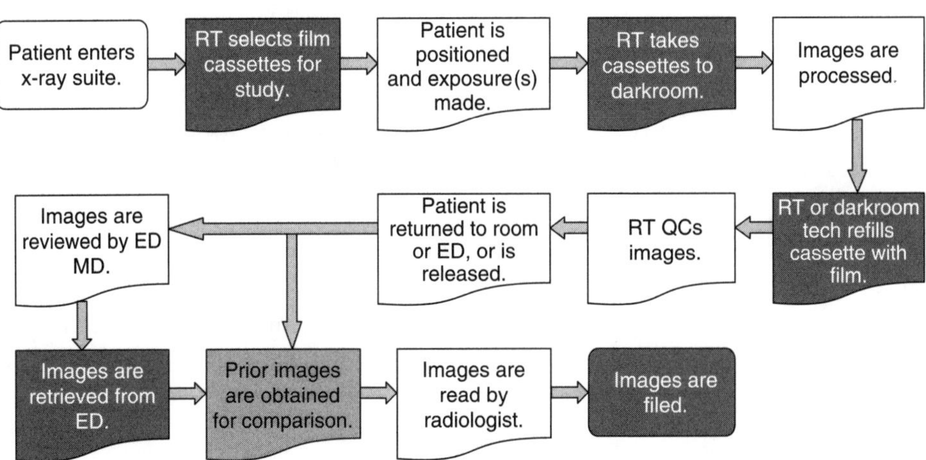

Figure 12.3 Digital radiography process changes RT indicates radiology technologist; QC, quality control; ED, emergency department; MD, doctor of medicine. Functions no longer necessary are highlighted in light gray. Functions performed electronically are highlighted in dark gray.

In addition to these aspects of the analysis, Step 4 will also include an overview of implementation. This overview should include personnel training concerns, network infrastructure upgrades, and the timeline necessary for those upgrades. For example, if the current network infrastructure is configured with 10-Mbps switches and the new network needs 100-Mbps switches to support the information flow, who will be responsible for managing this piece of the project, how will it be accomplished, and what is a reasonable timeline to expect it to be finished?

Financing Options and Benchmarking

Radiology administrators have historically been scrupulous about where their dollars are allocated, but never more so than in today's highly intensive capital technology investments, such as PACS, RIS, and digital radiographic equipment. Depending on the scope of the project, most CFOs believe that a return on investment of 3 to 5 years is necessary to pay off a project—that is, to recoup the initial investment—while generating enough passive income to support a profit stream for a determinable number of years after the break-even point. As such, radiology administrators are held accountable for trimming operating costs annually by managing their resources through an operating budget to improve the return on investment on the initial capital outlay for large projects, such as PACS.

An example of a return on investment using the previous year's expenses as a benchmark follows. Say a facility expended $1 million on film costs in the last fiscal year. The radiology administrator provides a financial proforma demonstrating the initial capital outlay while illustrating a reduction in operational expenses by reducing film cost by 50%, or $500,000, the following year. This 50% reduction in film costs can assist in the return on investment by eliminating the redundant cost of film and digital storage of images, in addition to lessening the length of time for the payback or break-even point on the initial investment. The benchmark of the prior year's expenses serves as the milestone to measure against for this year's expenses on film.

The hospital radiology administrator who is competing with other hospital or organizational profit centers for the same internal capital dollars has several options to consider for acquiring capital-intensive technology or equipment, such as PACS. Two options are purchase and lease. A third option is to forgo acquisition and use an application service provider.

Depending on the type of organization, the outlook for purchasing capital equipment will be different. Large organizations usually make outright purchases of equipment, dependent on cash flow and financial cash on hand for outright purchases. Imaging centers tend to lease equipment, requiring less startup cash and allowing for the equipment to be installed and revenue to be generated. Leases may be long or short term. Short-terms leases, such as leases of 1 to 2 years, are desirable when the organization believes it will soon secure funding for an outright purchase of the equipment or when capital funding is restricted or unavailable.

An organization of any size may use an application service provider. The financial benchmarks of previous years can assist with the forecasting of financial success in determining how to best finance the cost of the capital project and the project's net return on investment.

Financial Analysis

The most common types of financial analysis for CFOs to use for capital expenditures are payback period (PBP) analysis, net present value (NPV) analysis, rate of return (ROR) analysis, and internal rate of return (IRR) analysis. It is important for the radiology administrator to have a basic understanding of these four common analysis models.

PBP analysis determines the number of years required for cashflows to recover the original investment (or capital outlay):

$$\text{Payback period} = \text{Initial investment}/\text{Annual benefits}$$

The PBP analysis is easy to use compared with the other options. However, it is not the most accurate because PBP analysis does not take into account the effects of time on money. (It assumes no rate of inflation or opportunity for future investment income.) The PBP approach gives the radiology administrator a working timetable in terms of approximate months or actual years to payoff or break-even point on the investment.

NPV analysis identifies the value of the present-day investment dollars, using an estimate for inflation and valuation of the dollar, in future net cashflows, while deducting the original investment dollars:

$$\text{Net present value} = (\text{Cash flow} \times \text{Present value factor}) - \text{Investment amount}$$

The NPV analysis is commonly used for capital expenditures, as it provides the radiology administrator with an answer in future dollar amounts. The PBP analysis, in contrast, gives the radiology administrator an answer in years.

SIDEBAR: Summary of Baseline Analysis

- *Baseline analysis* is documentation of the current situation as part of the strategic and tactical decision making necessary to implement any plan for the future. The development of a baseline analysis begins by documenting the current state and then using the current state as a benchmark for conducting a look-back.
- *SWOT analysis* identifies functions or tasks, as well as external factors such as competitors, market changes, population changes, etc as current strengths/weaknesses or opportunities/threats.
- *Subjective information* is perceived to be fact but is unverified and unvalidated.
- *Objective information* is quantified or measured as a definable fact that has been verified and validated.
- *Baseline analysis* is a four-step plan of action:

  Step 1. Establish a goal and benchmark.
  Step 2. Record and organize the existing operational workflow.
  Step 3. Diagram the current state of operational systems.
  Step 4. Diagram the projected state of systems (where the facility wants to be), and identify steps (plan of action, strategy, and tactics) necessary to get from the current state to the projected state.

- In *financial analysis benchmarking,* the benchmark of the prior year's expenses serves as the milestone to measure against this year's expenses.
- *Payback period (PBP) analysis* determines the number of years required for cashflows to recover the original investment (or capital outlay):

  Payback period = Initial investment/Annual benefits

  The PBP approach gives the radiology administrator a working timetable in terms of approximate months or actual years to payoff or break-even point on the investment.
- *Net present value (NPV) analysis* determines the value of the present-day investment dollars, using an estimate for inflation and valuation of the dollar, in future net cashflows, while deducting the original investment dollars:

  Net present value = (Cash flow × Present value) − Investment amount

  The NPV analysis is a commonly used process for capital expenditures, as it provides the radiology administrator an answer in future dollar amounts.
- *Rate of return (ROR) analysis* shows the amount of financial return on a project, divided by the total amount invested:

  Rate of return = Amount of return/Amount of investment

- *Internal Rate of Return (IRR)* is the discount rate of a capital expense, where the discounted cashflows equal the original expense of the investment. The IRR analysis provides the radiology administrator an answer in terms of percentage.

ROR analysis shows the amount of financial return on a project, divided by the total amount invested. This analysis is the simplest (least cumbersome) to calculate, but it is typically only a quick estimate and is not thoroughly reliable:

Rate of return = Amount of return / Amount of investment

The IRR is the discount rate of a capital expense, where the discounted cashflows equal the original expense of the investment. Whereas the NPV analysis gives the radiology administrator an answer in dollars and the PBP analysis gives an answer in time, the IRR analysis provides an answer in terms of percentage. The calculations used to derive this analysis are cumbersome and typically require a computerized calculator.

Defining Success

No baseline analysis performed for a change in technology will be truly complete without some measure of postimplementation success. What expectations will be used to define this success? The leadership of most organizations will expect the radiology administrator to be able not just to define how to measure the success of the project but also to quantify those successes at predefined intervals after the initial implementation.

The radiology environment yields many possibilities for evaluation measures to determine the success of the project. A wide variety of variables can be identified or even combined to serve as success indicators:

- Does the new technology give the facility more name recognition in the marketplace?
- Has the new technology improved patient care or improved the patient experience (for example, reduced errors, reduced repeated studies, or improved customer satisfaction)?
- Has the new technology improved the mission of the organization (for example, improved regulatory compliance, increased productivity, or reduced costs)?
- Has the new technology created a solution—either short or long term—to a continuing problem (for example, improved recruitment, reduced turnover, or reduced lost images)?

For a long-term project such as the implementation of a PACS program, success benchmarks should be established as part of the benchmark analysis. These benchmarks must reflect specific time intervals not only during the project but also at project completion and at 3 months, 6 months, and 12 months following the completion of the project.

Conclusion

A baseline analysis should be a functional part of any technology evaluation for radiology administrators and for each supervisor whose job function adds to or detracts from the success of the radiology administrator. Open interviews with section supervisors and division managers not only establish open communication and trust but also yield the most current information on how the new technology will affect facility operations. The verbal interview process provides subjective information. Using the other aspects of the baseline analysis, the radiology administrator is able to correlate the subjective with the objective information to see if the proposed technology changes truly have the potential to help the facility reach the desired goal or resolve the problem. Use of the four-step process will help to establish operation benchmarks for years to come and allow the radiology administrator to better contend with operational changes when required to make them.

Most imaging or radiology facility administrators must make recommendations or technology decisions that sometimes are outside their area of expertise or influence to complete a task or job assigned to them. When applying the skills learned from this chapter regarding the understanding and application of a baseline analysis and while incorporating strong financial analysis, the radiology administrator will be better prepared to handle a look-back at projects and to make future forecasts for operational improvements.

Chapter 13

Information Technology in Imaging: The Value-Driven Approach

Deniese M. Chaney

The dependency on IT in radiology has increased dramatically with the advent of improved image processing and computer-aided diagnosis, as well as the demand for greater specificity in the documentation of quality and outcomes. However, the use of these technologies is far from universal, and the techniques are implemented with varying results. The cost of these systems has slowed their adoption, but the lack of perceived or real value received from implementations has also contributed. This chapter offers approaches to improving the success of radiology IT projects. It describes how to plan for radiology IT and then select and implement it to provide the maximum benefit to the facility and the maximum impact on the quality of services delivered to customers.

General access to health data has been on organizational agendas for many years, but realization of the goal has been illusive.[1,2] Healthcare delivery systems around the world have begun developing the electronic medical record (EMR). Past generations of these systems were known as the hospital information systems (HIS) or clinical information systems (CIS) and comprised the clinical workflow systems, financial systems, supply management systems, and clinical documentation systems.

Radiology information (patient history, reports, and images) is important to achieving the goal of electronic data availability regardless of physical location. Although there are major hurdles to overcome to achieve broad adoption across the industry, both the government and healthcare delivery organizations are actively pursuing solutions to infrastructure, standardization of data, and patient access to information issues.[3-5] As a future contributor to, and consumer of, EMRs, radiology facilities should begin planning their IT with global electronic data access in mind. This chapter includes some methods for incorporating these future needs into the planning, selection, implementation, and use of the RIS and PACS.

Huang[6] defines both RIS and PACS systems in *PACS and Imaging Informatics: Basic Principles and Applications*. This text presents a detailed examination of the components and function of PACS, its integration with RIS and other systems, and its use in clinical practice today. RIS and PACS are defined as follows:

- *RIS*. "The RIS is designed to support both the administrative and clinical operation of a radiology department, to reduce administrative overhead, and to improve the quality of radiological examination delivery."[6] RIS systems have proved their value to the clinical and financial function of radiology departments by flagging and reporting incomplete process queues (such as examinations with no report and dictated examinations with no transcription), automating and standardizing the charge capture and billing process, providing data to allow improvements in overall procedure turnaround time, and managing equipment resource scheduling and staffing.
- *PACS*. "A picture archiving and communication system consists of image and data acquisition, storage and display subsystems integrated by digital networks and application software. It can be as simple as a film digitizer connected to a display workstation with a small image database or as complex as an enterprise image management system."[6] PACS, first developed in the late 1980s for electronic radiology imaging, has become increasingly important in the practice of medical imaging across many specialties. These complex IT systems have greatly improved access to imaging information across the clinical enterprise, improved radiology turnaround time, reduced study retake rates, greatly reduced the number of unread cases, and improved the quality and speed of image interpretation.

Dictation systems that support radiology reporting have been in general use for many years. These systems provide a centralized electronic means for generating digital voice recording of reports. Dictation systems are interfaced to RIS and often to PACS to enable linking of the right examination with the dictation and the transcribed result. By using these systems with the proper interfaces, radiologists can be assured that their dictations are attached to the right examination, thus reducing errors.

Transcriptionists use the system to listen to and type the radiology report into the RIS, providing a human interface between the dictation system and the RIS results module. Radiology management can use the reports generated from these systems to track transcription turnaround, transcriptionist productivity, and the backlog of untranscribed minutes of dictation. The findings provide consistent data for staffing the transcription function based on the volume of work. Later generations of dictation systems—speech or voice recognition technology—have also been generally available for use in radiology for a number of years. Speech systems have been marketed as reducing the cost of radiology operations by eliminating the radiology transcription function. However, overworked radiologists have been reluctant to spend the time required to train on the systems and to take the responsibility for editing their own reports when the transcription function is eliminated. This reluctance has slowed the implementation of speech recognition systems in general or limited their use where they have been implemented. As a result, careful planning and a high level of commitment from radiologists should be in place before making these budgetary commitments.

The clinical benefits of using speech recognition can be measured in significant reductions in report turnaround time that translate into more timely information to support clinical decisions. This enhanced service can increase clinician loyalty and provide a competitive advantage for a radiology facility.[7] In the longer term, the use of speech recognition can reduce the overall cost of care and reduce lengths of stay if clinicians can take advantage of the results more quickly.

Getting Value from IT Investments

Many radiology IT system projects start with vendor selection, followed by system installation mostly driven by the vendor. The organization often does not take the opportunity to make improvements to the clinical and business processes enabled by the new system or undertake the advance planning required to take full advantage of the system capabilities. The old adage still applies: An information system layered on top of a bad manual process will only make the problems with the manual system more glaring. Implementing a great system into a poorly designed manual operation will make the process problems more apparent, do nothing to resolve them, and increase the workload of the people using the system. Increasing the value achieved from IT requires investment—investment in structuring the project for success and getting the right people involved early; investment in understanding the needs of the organization and selecting a vendor to meet those needs, matching system capabilities with planned operations improvements; and investment in actively managing the project beginning to end.[8]

In the following three scenarios, *value* is defined as both the functional and operational benefit of a systems implementation, and *investment* is defined as the level of organizational commitment and the time and money expenditure necessary to ensure that value is achieved. Figure 13.1 illustrates the value an organization can expect to achieve for different levels of investment. There is some minimal value derived from any IT project. The RIS, for example, will organize the reporting process and provide

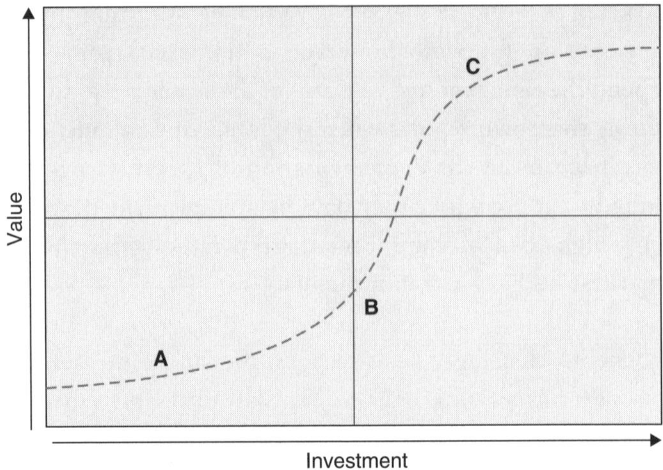

Figure 13.1 Value-investment curve: the value an organization can expect to achieve for different levels of investment The dotted line represents the value curve.

automatic tracking and reporting features not available to a manual operation. There are also levels of investment after which marginal value can be achieved. As a result, the value derived will always be more than 0% and rarely, if ever, 100%. The dotted line in Figure 13.1 shows that the value derived will increase rapidly for incremental investments after a certain point and level off as it approaches maximum value. The goal is to achieve the most value and maximize the investment, putting the organization in the upper right quadrant of the graph, near the peak of the curve.

At point A in Figure 13.1, the organization and the vendor invest little in the project and achieve little value. This scenario can sometimes occur in application service provider (ASP) implementations in which the vendor's revenues are dependent upon going live. The vendor minimizes the cost of the implementation, and the organization assumes that minimal structure and investment are required as well. Transformational change of clinical and business processes is not undertaken or is undertaken only at a minimal level. The result is that little real organizational value is derived from the investment.

At point B in Figure 13.1, the organization starts the project with a vendor selection and then pays the vendor a lot of money to implement the system. This approach results in minimal investment in internal project structure, project planning, and broad-based organizational commitment. Some vendors offer rudimentary workflow analysis services with this level of investment, but the organization is rarely prepared to adopt even these minimal changes because the information is available too late in the process. Once the system implementation begins, all the attention and resources will be focused on technical aspects. The result will be an expensive system implementation with little organizational value.

At point C in Figure 13.1, the organization commits the time and resources early enough in the project to affect the project's overall conduct. The investment in time, resources, and money is significantly higher than in the first two scenarios, but the value achieved is also significantly greater. The value an organization expects to receive from radiology IT projects must be defined and metrics aligned with the components of the value statement. As a result, the value achieved will vary by organization and cannot be universally defined. Establishing a threshold of expectation will provide a target for the project team and start the project down the road to a successful conclusion. However, setting expectations alone will not ensure success. The balance of this chapter is devoted to describing the structure, process, and commitment required to achieve greater value from IT investments.

IT Procurement Challenge

Whether the facility is considering its first IT procurement or is an experienced buyer of RIS or PACS, the procurement process for IT products and services should be structured and consistent with the longer-range goals for the organization in which it will be implemented.

Organizations considering IT procurements should also review their options for merging the functions of a number of the workflow systems used. These mergers are accomplished through either system-to-system interfaces (codified by data exchange between systems but little or no ability to interact with system functionality except in the native system) or system integrations (real system interactions are enabled in either of the integrated systems to appear seamless to the user). Radiology facilities that use RIS, PACS, or dictation/speech recognition systems should evaluate the options available from the vendors for tightly merging the functions of any or all these systems with the new procurement. Because of the workflow improvements and time savings possible when system integrations are deployed, they should be seriously considered with any new IT procurement for radiology.

Getting Organized and Developing the
Project Strategy and Scope

When it comes to the process by which IT systems are selected, organizations should give considerable thought to why the system under consideration would be beneficial. Organizations should understand the problems the system is expected to solve, the groups the system will serve, and the way the system will be supported after it is implemented. To accomplish these tasks, it is critical to involve the right people in making the decisions that will guide the project and engaging that group in developing and prioritizing the needs and selection criteria, developing the scope of the project, and devising the implementation strategy. Throughout the project planning, procurement, and implementation, the system owners, technical support team, and systems administrators should be defining and refining the operations and support model for the system after going live.

The first objective of any major RIS or PACS project should be to identify the right project sponsor and executive decision-making team to guide the project. Ideally, the project sponsor will have significant influence over the approval and funding of the project and be committed to participating in the planning and decision making. The project sponsor will be a member of the executive steering team for the project.

The executive steering team will be involved in decision making for the project. The makeup of this group is slightly different for each organization and will vary by system type (RIS or PACS), but involving key stakeholders early in the process will greatly improve the success of the project. It is important to include institutional leadership, IT experts, customers, key radiologist stakeholders, and user groups. Input from key imaging customer groups (intensive users of imaging services) is critical to designing a PACS implementation to improve the quality of services delivered to these customers. Incorporating these customers into the strategy and design of the system implementation (as it affects their practice) will improve the chances that these customers will both understand and support the capabilities of the system being implemented and make use of it in their clinical practices.

A PACS project should be planned for the radiology facility somewhat differently than general and key customer access to images and other patient information, though the two efforts must be coordinated to minimize conflicts or overlap. The RIS project should be planned jointly with IT to ensure that clinical data are available to the RIS for radiology use and that status updates and results are available to clinical services. If an EMR strategy has been developed for the organization, the radiology department should make sure its plans are aligned and complementary.

The working groups (organized by major categories of work) are the key task teams for the project. These groups should be made up of representatives of users affected by the implementation and be charged with participating in the planning, design, and implementation of the system. These groups remain consistent throughout the project and report to the executive steering team both the status of the project and any progress issues. In most projects, there should be major categories of work in the following areas:

- A clinical team focused on clinical process needs and workflow redesign.
- A technical team focused on system interactions, including interfaces, network infrastructure, data center requirements, and system support after going live.
- In a PACS project, an enterprise key stakeholder team that will focus on the special needs and system design for clinical users of electronic images across the enterprise.
- A project management designee or project management office to oversee the work of all the working groups and report status to the executive steering team.

The project structure provides the framework and resources to manage the project according to the plans that will be developed.

Once the executive steering team and working groups are organized and chartered, these groups should start the development of the strategy and scope of the project by completing the following activities:

1. Make a list of goals for the project, outlining major clinical and business objectives and the project approval process to be used. Each organization will have programmatic plans to which RIS or PACS might be applied. The organization might be planning a business expansion for radiology, and RIS or PACS could enable more efficient operations. The executive sponsor should be able to assist in gathering the information required to determine the approval process for the project; the timelines required for leadership review; and if needed, the board presentation requirements.

2. Perform a needs assessment that defines the clinical and business problems the system is expected to resolve. A good place to start is where the organization now experiences the most difficulty in aspects such as workflow, lost charges, and dropped processes. For example, would it be advantageous if the system supported such functions as emergency department discordance tracking/resolution, urgent results messaging, urgent results communication tracking, and voice clips? If the organization already has RIS or PACS, it is a good idea to incorporate the gaps or unmet needs in the current system. The needs assessment should consider future needs for new technology, programmatic expansion, and external business opportunities for both radiology and its customers. For radiology, include nuclear medicine, ultrasonography with or without three- or four-dimensional (motion) capability, digital mammography, three-dimensional reconstruction, speech recognition, or other subsystem needs.

For customers, the needs assessment should include a list of subsystems and requirements for other image-generating services such as cardiology, radiation oncology, ophthalmology, dermatology, and gastrointestinal medicine. Finally, the team should determine whether it would be advantageous to have these subsystems and the RIS or other workflow systems be fully integrated and whether the integration plan would change the vendor qualification criteria.[9] The decisions made now about the level of product integration will affect the initial and long-term costs of the project and the pool of vendors to be considered, so it's a good idea to carefully evaluate options now. The resulting needs list provides a partial list of functional requirements for the system and the major vendor selection criteria for the system. The selection criteria should be prioritized and weighted for use in evaluating vendor responses.

3. Define an implementation scope and strategy to provide initial inputs for the institutional portion of the project plan. The implementation scope establishes the phasing and timing of the implementation; it determines for whom and when. At the conclusion of the strategy phase, the team will have the high-level information needed to develop an initial project time line using this information.

4. Develop a strategy for conformance to the organization's EMR strategy (or enterprise distribution, if no EMR strategy exists). The goal of this development should be simply to eliminate data silos and barriers to clinical user single point of access to data. Data silos are created when interfaces have to provide the connectivity between disparate systems and data. A good rule of thumb to use when planning systems is that wherever data silos exist, barriers to access will follow (see the Sidebar).

5. Conduct an initial review of the vendor community to establish a list of qualified vendors that have the potential to serve the organization. At this point in the process, informal data gathering should suffice to determine if there are major issues that would prevent a vendor from being considered.

SIDEBAR: EMR Implementations

Few EMR implementations are without some interfaces to disparate systems, but these interfaces should be minimized. The EMR is usually implemented to provide hospital-based clinicians and most external constituents with a single point for access to all data. By eliminating data silos for IT systems used by radiology and other image-generating services, the organization (in collaborative discussions with IT staff and key stakeholders) will establish system requirements for image and results access through the EMR. The functional requirements for general enterprise access and access of key specialty users should emerge from this task and be added to the functional requirements and vendor selection criteria.

Published data are available from organizations such as Gartner and rating surveys from KLAS that could supply the organization with a starting point. However, every organization is unique in some areas, and the market is changing rapidly enough to require a fresh investigation of the market at this point in the process. It will be important to gather the following types of information about the vendor's current offering:

- System architecture requirements and compliance with institutional network and hardware standards.
- Information about compliance with institutional IT standards.
- Database and application structures.
- Information on the standard user interface.
- Current system features and functions.

The formal process to evaluate vendors will be discussed later. At the conclusion of this initial review, the plan should be to limit the vendor pool to no more than five vendors to be included in the formal review. It may be necessary to conduct more research and submit a request for information if a larger vendor list persists after additional discussion. This process will add considerable time to the vendor evaluation but can save time later in the formal vendor evaluation.

6. Document current state process flows. Begin discussing the challenges imposed with the current processes and desired outcomes from the radiology IT project.

Vendor Evaluation

Preparing to Bid: Development of the RFP, Pricing Configuration, and Attachments

The goal of conducting a vendor evaluation should be to determine the gap between institutional needs and the vendor's capabilities, as well as to determine the organizational value to be derived from the required investment. Now that the organization has defined the scope and direction of the project and its functional needs, the process of evaluating the qualified vendors can begin.

This process should be as objective as possible, allowing a direct comparison of the vendors rather than open-ended request for proposal (RFP) questions. Develop specific statements demonstrating the technical and clinical needs defined earlier as a starting point, and build the vendor inquiry from that point forward. Consider using a yes/no or scored format as a way to clearly obtain an "apples-to-apples" vendor comparison. Table 13.1 shows examples of inquiries that fit this criterion.

Vendors should receive a structured pricing configuration so that initial price quotes are meaningful for comparison purposes. The level of detail typically submitted by

Table 13.1 Sections from Sample Vendor Inquiry

		Question Type	No = 0 Yes = 3 Scale: 0-4	Comments
2	Experience with buyer, current information systems, and site visit proposal		N/A	See Client Operating Environment File
	2.1 Vendor has implemented and provided a bi-directional interface with vendor's PACS product and buyer's RIS	Y/N		See Client Operating Environment File
	2.2 Vendor has implemented and provided clinician interface through buyer's clinical information system vendor	Y/N		See Client Operating Environment File
	2.3 Please propose a site visit candidate for buyer if vendor is included in the finalists for the selection. Preferably this site will have the buyer's RIS and clinicals with integration to digital dictation/speech recognition and all system features offered by the vendor	Text	N/A	See Client Operating Environment File
	1.3 Image retrieval and display			
	1.3.1 Application manages images and displays images from all imaging types listed above in a consistent manner regardless of user type (radiologist, technologist, referring MD) or workstation configuration (as long as the workstation configuration meets minimum specifications defined)	Y/N		
	1.3.2 Application supports real-time ultrasound viewing and raw data storage, doppler, and sound	Y/N		Describe any exceptions
	1.3.3 Application supports nuclear medicine image analysis and processing and raw data storage	Y/N		If no, how are nuclear medicine readings accomplished?
	1.3.4 Application supports PET image processing and image fusion	Y/N		If no, how are PET readings accomplished?
	1.3.5 Application supports radiation oncology portal imaging and direct export of data to treatment planning systems	Y/N		If no, how is radiation oncology data managed?
	1.3.6 Application supports full-fidelity digital mammography image processing and viewing	Y/N		If no, how are digital mammography readings accomplished?
	1.3.7 Application supports cardiac catheterization image management and viewing, including cine	Y/N		If no, how are cardiac cath readings accomplished?
	1.3.7.1 Application can capture and store cardiac images from the system at the buyer's site	Y/N		See Client Operating Environment file for support data
	1.3.8 Proposed system supports 3D and 4D ultrasound image retrieval and display with color	Y/N		

	1.3.9	Proposed system supports retrieval and display of volumetric data	Y/N		Describe the uses employed in proposed system
	1.3.10	Image retrieval and display are consistent across all acquisition modalities, and work can commence on data sets prior to fully loading large studies (ie, streamed data)	Y/N		If no, explain the impact of modality type on retrieval and display of images
	1.3.11	Radiology reports are viewed on the PACS monitors OR on a separate monitor and are buyer configurable	Y/N		
	1.3.12	Image scrolling (on fully loaded data sets) is smooth and does not require pauses while the system "catches up with the user"	Y/N		
	1.3.13	Vendor has integrated the buyer's 3D reconstruction vendor applications in at least one site	Y/N		See Client Operating Environment file for support data
	1.3.14	Proposed system application offers MPR/3D reconstruction tools for all authorized users and system stores and retrieves reconstructed files and movies	Y/N		Briefly describe tools used

vendors at this stage is too limited to be of real value and often creates more questions about what is or is not included in the bid than it answers. Therefore, the objective of providing a structured pricing configuration is to eliminate most of the questions about what is included in the vendor's price and to provide the organization with the ability to cross-compare the vendor responses more directly. Vendors should be asked to provide list pricing and discounted pricing for the specified configuration. Because the vendor of choice will need to configure the system specifically for the organization as a part of final negotiations, a preliminary specification should suffice for the initial bid. Table 13.2 is a section of a price specification document showing some of the items that could be included. Typically, the vendor will be asked to bid the main system components, peripheral devices, core application software licenses, and other needed application modules. Initial implementation costs, training, and maintenance should be bid separately in the event the organization will separate what would typically be operating costs from the capital investments in the system.

If the vendors under consideration are not known to the stakeholders, it might help to require the vendors to participate in on-site scripted demonstrations during the response period. Doing so will provide interested parties with an opportunity to engage the vendors in discussions specific to their needs before the evaluation advances to the

Table 13.2 Sample Pricing Section

Directions for Completing Pricing Sheets						
General Instructions: The configuration supplied in this document is a straw system configuration ONLY and is intended to provide a framework for comparison of vendor prices. A final configuration for the systems to be supplied will be determined with the vendor of choice during contract negotiations. Unit prices will, however, be binding. Therefore, it is critical that each bidder provide unit prices and committed discounts at the unit price level.						
Category	*Buyer's Component Description*	*Quantity*	*Vendor's Component Description*	*Part Number*	*Unit List Price*	*Extended List Price*
Core PACS Application Software Licenses						
Bidder will quote quantity where applicable (site license is preferable wherever possible for all applications). Please detail any additional functionality included in the core application (ie, MPR, 3D, mini-PACS capability, etc). Please refer to the Client Operating Environment File for procedure volume projections by site and for the enterprise.						
APP	Core PACS Application Software	1			—	—
APP	Diagnostic Radiology User Licenses	10			—	—
Total Core PACS Application Software Licenses						$—
Enterprise Concurrent User Licenses (if priced separately)						
ENT ACC	Clinician (non-Radiology) enterprise site license	1			—	—
ENT ACC	Alternate proposal for enterprise licensing– include license numbers for 200 concurrent users as an example and how vendor would price incremental packages	0			—	—
Total Enterprise Concurrent User Licenses (if priced separately)						$—
Data Conversion						
Bidders are asked to provide a cost for converting existing electronic PACS image and database files to the new system as a means to avoid parallel systems. Please see the Client Environment file for the information needed to complete this section.						
IMAGE CONV	Specify pricing to convert the existing legacy image files into the new PACS solution				—	—
DBMS CONV	Specify pricing to convert the existing PACS DBMS data into the new PACS solution				—	—

RIS PT HX CONV	Specify pricing to load RIS patient history into the new PACS				—	—
OTHER	Specify other pricing needed to complete the data conversion				—	—
Total Data Conversion						—
Required Hardware						
HW	Specify any hardware required for the recommended configuration that can only be supplied by the bidder specify quanties for each item separately and pricing	0			—	—
HW	Specify any hardware required for the recommended configuration that can only be supplied by the bidder—specify quanties for each item separately and pricing	0			—	—
Total Required Hardware						$—
Referring Clinician Modules						
Bidder will provide licensing information for any specialty software modules offered for referring clinicians. Please quote 1 each at this time. These modules are referenced in the Technical Requirements Document and address image processing and storage for clinical use (total joint surgical planning for Orthopedics, surgical planning for Neurosurgeons, Cardiac Cath, etc).						
REF CLIN	Describe module and bid one license unless there are price breaks for concurrent users—then bid one concurrent user quantity	0			—	—
REF CLIN	Describe module and bid one license unless there are price breaks for concurrent users then bid one concurrent user quantity	0			—	—
Total Referring Clinician Modules						$—

formal review of written responses. It is typical to allow 3 weeks for vendor responses to a structured written inquiry. Depending on the number of vendors under evaluation, the scripted demonstrations could add 1 to 2 weeks to the process but would provide an initial understanding of the vendors' approach and product offerings.

If scripted demonstrations are being used, schedule each vendor to bring in a system or systems, and provide a detailed clinical scenario that each vendor must use for the demonstration. Schedule a separate demonstration period (a full day, if possible) for each vendor, and run the demonstrations several times to allow adequate opportunities for evaluators to participate. The objective of these demonstrations is to acquaint the decision makers with each of the vendors—nothing more. The clinical scenario should be designed to elicit information about some of the organization's most complex challenges. The vendors' preparation and capability will become evident in both the way they respond to the clinical scenario and the amount of information they share about their approach during the demonstrations. Vendors should be required to submit a recent financial statement, a sample implementation project plan, a description of the requirements for the organization's systems administrator, and any other subsidiary information required by the organization.

Releasing the Bid Package

Now that the organization has accumulated the information needed from the vendors, it will be necessary to prepare a cover document that describes the sections of the bid, the attachments, the response requirements, the deadline for the response, the response format (electronic format, hard copy, or both), and any regulatory compliance requirements. If a prebid conference is required, the schedule and details should be included. It is also appropriate to require vendors to submit a formal notification-of-intent-to-respond form within a week of the bid release to signify their interest in being included in the solicitation. See Table 13.3 for a bid attachment checklist.

It is typical to release these packages electronically, so it will be necessary to obtain the correct contact information for the vendors. This is also a good time to schedule the vendors for scripted demonstrations and prepare them for receipt of the package. After the bid package is released and vendors have confirmed receipt, designated individuals should be available to answer general questions from the bidders.

During the response period, prepare the evaluation forms that will be used to score the vendor responses. Pull out all the documents developed up to this point, and develop a scoring instrument to cover all the goals, needs, selection criteria, and

Table 13.3 Bid Attachment Checklist

Item	Description
Operating environment	Consider the following: network topology; hardware vendor limitations; database preferences; interface/integration systems and standards supported; system backup standards; and storage architecture requirements, including whether the data from the new system will be stored on existing or new systems.
Procedure volumes	Develop a multiyear projection of procedure volumes by modality for radiology and cumulatively for other image-generating services to be included in the bid.
Demonstration script	This is the clinical scenario that will be used for the on-site scripted demonstrations, if they are used.
Modality equipment list (PACS)	If this is a PACS evaluation, include a list of the equipment that will be attached to the system. Include the modality vendor, the date of acquisition and last upgrade, the current software release (if applicable), and DICOM conformance if it is known. The vendor will use this information to quote the interfaces between the modalities and the PACS.
Selection criteria:	
†References	The vendor should provide a list of "like" references with the appropriate contact people in the organization who can be called to obtain direct input on the vendor's performance. Provide the criteria to be met by the vendor in selecting the references.
†Location for site visit	If the vendor were included in the finalists, what site would be selected for an on-site visit? Provide the criteria to be met by the vendor in selecting the site.

†Items that must be completed and returned by the vendor with the bid package.

inquiries included in the bid package. The formal evaluation of the responses will form one of several inputs to the final vendor selection process. Other inputs are discussed in later sections.

Evaluating the Responses

The evaluation of the responses is where all the advance work pays off. If the bid documents and evaluation forms have been structured correctly, the evaluation team can focus on the content of the responses rather than the structure of the evaluation. The evaluators will spend considerable time reviewing the responses, so it is important to take best advantage of their input. Organize the review so that each evaluator has the opportunity to read and score each response, because the objective at this point is to compare qualified vendors. One way to minimize the time required of each evaluator is to divide the reviews by section. For example, the IT team should evaluate the IT sections of the responses; the radiologists, technologists, nurses, and clerks the clinical sections and any specific functionality requirements for radiology; and so forth. Clinical stakeholders should review sections corresponding to their clinical and technical needs. However, any evaluator should be able to score the entire response if desired. The greater the shared knowledge generated during the formal evaluation, the better the decision making. Remember, these procurements create long-term relationships with a company and its products. The finance department should review the financial reports and provide a summary of the company's financial history and any potential risks posed by a long-term relationship with the vendor.

To evaluate the pricing proposals, tabulate the responses in a comparison format for now, and develop an initial project life cycle cost using preliminary pricing from each vendor. It will be important to develop a multiyear cost projection for the system that also includes any new staffing needs as a part of the budgetary recommendation for the project. The life cycle cost of a major radiology IT project is high and will likely compete with other IT initiatives within the organization. As a result, a return on investment analysis is sometimes required. The details behind this analysis are not discussed here, but it is important to know that some leadership and board packages will require such analysis. When a return on investment analysis is required, the organization will often have an approved format for use in accumulating such things as costs, revenues, and cost reduction commitments (see the Sidebar).

Depending on the procurement strategy—capital purchase or operational payments (ASPs)—the major components of the cost will add up on either the capital or operating side of the analysis. It is common for the entire evaluation process to take several weeks and to accumulate a volume of data to be carried forward to the next evaluation phase.

Narrowing the Vendor Pool

The team now has a pool of objective information about each vendor and a set of organization-specific weighted selection criteria, needs, and goals. The next step is to eliminate those vendors unlikely to fulfill the breadth and depth of the organizational need. Prepare a summary of the weighted scores for each vendor, financial evaluation documents, and any conclusions drawn from the response evaluations

---

SIDEBAR: Life Cycle Costs

The life cycle costs of RIS or PACS projects are the cumulative capital and operating costs of the project for the life of the system. Consider the following formula:

Life cycle costs = (Capital investment required to keep the system current for each of
7 years) + (Maintenance and other operating costs of the system for 7 years).

Note: Seven years is assumed to be the life of the system in this illustration.

---

for review by the executive steering team, the working groups, and key stakeholders. The goal of this phase is to narrow the pool of vendors to no more than three for site visits. Getting to three vendors may take several rounds of discussion with the groups. The weighted selection criteria should provide a structure for achieving consensus on many of the major items. The political and relationship items will also become apparent at this stage, so it is important to anticipate them and factor them into the process; be sure to determine how much weight will be given to these items. If necessary, segment the consensus sessions by selection criteria item and gain support item by item until the list of remaining items is small enough to allow discussion of a mechanism to achieve consensus on the remaining open items.

The vendor finalists should be notified immediately to prepare for site visits, because scheduling the site visit team and the site can take 3 to 4 weeks. Schedules must be cleared, and vendors must make sure the appropriate people are available for the site visit.

Visiting the Site and Naming Finalists

Prepare for the site visits by accumulating a list of unanswered questions or gaps in the vendor evaluation up to this point. The list should be somewhat different for each vendor and can be converted into a scoring tool or simply used to guide the items to be covered on the day of the visit. However, it will be important to capture the information gathered on the site visits as inputs to the final phase in the vendor evaluation—naming the two finalists. Use the same processes that worked in the vendor evaluation phase to narrow the pool of candidates following site visits and name the finalists.

There is much debate about how to handle the vendor interactions at this point. One school of thought is to have two vendors involved (ranked equally) to provide the organization additional leverage in negotiating the business and contractual terms. This method is appropriate if both vendors could provide a suitable solution and the organization was prepared to negotiate with either vendor. The second school of thought is to negotiate in good faith with the vendor ranked first among the two to yield a better business result. The choice of negotiating strategy is often determined by the team designated to negotiate, but favorable results are possible in either situation. It is now time to designate the negotiating team and move into contract negotiations.

Negotiating the Contract

Contract negotiations must be conducted openly and fairly. The goal of a good negotiation is to sign an agreement that both parties will support aggressively for the entire term of the relationship. This means that there can be no winner and no loser in the negotiation of terms and conditions. If the organization has a standard

IT agreement, it is recommended that it be used as the basis for beginning the discussions. If not, start with the vendor's standard IT agreement. Either way, work will be required to gain agreement on the document between the negotiating parties. ASP relationships require different contract vehicles than capital purchase agreements. Unless the organization has a history of developing contracts for ASP relationships, it is best to start with the vendor's contract. The only technique that should be avoided is use of a vendor's purchasing terms and conditions (the ones submitted when purchasing medical equipment) as a starting point for an IT relationship. These terms and conditions will not contain the depth of detailed terms needed to support both parties in a long-term relationship.

The vendor finalists should formally configure the system according to the needs specified by gathering additional information, coming on site to validate data, and meeting with the appropriate parties. This is a last chance to update the specifications for the quote before the final business terms (for example, pricing structure, pricing terms, guarantees, future discounts, and inclusions and exclusions) are negotiated. This is also the time to finalize the list of system interfaces and integrations to be included in the project, the services to be provided by the vendor in support of the implementation, the training program, and the service contract length and service level. The discount received in the formal response should be revisited and pricing agreed on now that the vendor is among the finalists.

It is common to designate a contract negotiations team of no more than four people, including the organization's attorney. Develop the contract draft to include those items important to the system relationship being negotiated. It will be important to incorporate specific future assurances agreed on during the business term negotiations and any special items affecting the long-term conduct of the relationship. Table 13.4 provides a reference list of some terms important to radiology IT contracts. Assuming the vendor is receiving the contract from the organization, the vendor should mark up the document (show the changes to the proposed terms) as appropriate and return it to the organization's attorney. The negotiating team should review the suggested changes from the vendor and initiate a call or face-to-face session or sessions to discuss the changes and agree on final terms. If both parties are negotiating in good faith, contract negotiations should not be protracted or difficult.

Most of the terms will be dictated by the standard agreement, and some will be added because of the nature of the relationship proposed. Be sure to take enough time preparing this document to ensure a good long-term working relationship with the vendor.

Table 13.4 Radiology-Specific Contract Terms Reference List

Item	Description
Service level agreements	These terms describe the overall performance of the system and penalties for nonperformance. They are typical in IT agreements.
System response time terms	These terms describe the committed response times for key functions in the system, such as display of the first image following an ad hoc query in PACS or presentation of a search result in RIS.
Service terms	These terms cover warranties, service response time, whether service will be provided on-site or off-site, any remote system monitoring, etc.
Implementation services terms	These terms should describe the services to be provided by the vendor and the organization during the implementation and ongoing system support. It is common to include them as an exhibit to the agreement.
System acceptance terms	These terms describe the condition of the system when it is accepted and ready for full clinical use. With phased implementation, the system is not fully implemented until the last phase is complete. It will be important to understand this fact when reviewing and agreeing to the acceptance, warranty, and first clinical use provisions in the agreement.
Termination terms	Although no one wants to work hard and end up having to terminate an agreement, it is important to have clearly understood conditions that would cause termination and to spell out the impact of the termination on both parties.
Obsolete hardware and refresh terms	These terms describe the provision for, and timing of, any committed hardware refresh; the consequences of obsolete hardware on the system; and the requirements of both parties in the event of occurrence.
Issues resolution after go-live terms	These terms describe the process to follow in resolving system issues that arise after go-live and the designated parties to be the point of contact for these activities.

Implementation

The media devoted to imaging are replete with articles describing radiology IT implementation experiences and methods. Less information is available about what affects implementation success. As discussed earlier, the organization's success criteria should be developed early in the process. Now is the time to plan the implementation to achieve the goals established during the strategy phase of the project. Implementation of radiology IT is usually complex and involves multiple constituents and multiple departments within the organization. Therefore, it is critical that the organization manage the overall project requirements, with the vendor acting as a major technical contributor to the project.

Getting Organized and Engaging the Vendor

The organization's project manager is responsible for coordinating across groups of constituents, phases of the project, and systems and subsystems being implemented. The individual or individuals in this role would ideally be involved in the project from the beginning, should be chosen carefully for the ability to manage complex projects, and should understand the systems being implemented. For radiology IT projects, clinical experience in imaging services is valuable and in some cases can be substituted for system understanding. Project management skills and experience are the most important, however. The person or persons being trained to take over the systems administration role following going live need to be incorporated into the project at this point so they may be trained during the implementation to begin taking over the system. If these individuals do not have experience in the role, it is unrealistic to expect them to be experts at go-live. They will require mentoring and support for a while to become fully effective.

The implementation working groups should include some individuals from the planning working groups to ensure continuity, and new members will be needed to handle new activities not yet undertaken. RIS and PACS projects often require a review of the network infrastructure for each of the vendor finalists, but the network enhancements defined earlier must now be implemented for the vendor of choice. For example, the demands of high-volume imaging with larger data sets (for example, CT or MRI studies of more than a thousand images or digital mammography) are placing new challenges on standard system architectures and networks. If the organization is incorporating these types of studies into the PACS, it would be advisable to conduct a review of the impact of these technologies on the network and server infrastructure for the new or existing PACS system.

The vendor should be able to provide a draft project plan and a staffing plan for the tasks to be undertaken by its project staff. The organization's project management should add the activities needed to complete the project plan, such as the following:

- The network enhancements discussed earlier.
- Data center improvements needed to host the system.
- Workflow analysis, redesign, and implementation.
- Organization-specific interface/integration activities, including designing to expose data and images from within the HIS/EMR and providing the radiology facility with information from the HIS/EMR. The vendor should supply its interface/integration methodology and tools for this effort and resources to begin the planning.

- System-specific activities in user areas such as renovations, furniture, and so on, and any approvals required to move forward with these changes.
- Input and output device planning and procurement if these devices are not supplied by the systems vendor (for example, data entry/data viewing and data distribution).
- The training master plan, including activities not supported by the vendor.
- The acceptance-testing algorithm and plan agreed upon in the contract.
- Project coordination, issues tracking, and risk management requirements across all constituencies, systems, subsystems, and project activities.

A project schedule will be developed and approved by the executive steering team. Project management is now ready to engage directly with the vendor to begin the implementation activities.

Coordinating the Project: Consolidated Project Plan

The vendor of choice for the IT project will focus its effort on the work that it must accomplish to implement the system. The radiology and IT departments must design the broader project plan to include both the vendor and the institutional requirements for the system implementation and all the precursors to enable the system to be successfully implemented within the organization. The requirements will vary by site, but an adequate master project plan will set expectations and over-all project requirements. It is important to spend sufficient effort developing the implementation plan so that overall workload and timelines are clearly understood by all key project constituents.

Workflow Transformation

Now that the vendor of choice is known, the organization can begin matching work-flow gaps and desired changes developed in the planning phase to the vendor's method of addressing those needs. The vendor should provide workflow experts from its team to address product capabilities to work with the organizational experts to design future processes and flows for patients and staff. This is also a good time to design paperless workflow, especially if the project involves incorporating PACS or dictation/speech recognition into a previously implemented RIS. Workflow trans-formation should have adequate resources to execute the changes within the timeline of the implementation. Change is the hardest thing to adopt in an IT project, but if the change actually improves the quality or timeliness of care delivered, it should be worth it. Therefore, changes must be designed to deliver results and include metrics to demonstrate the value achieved. The goals of a workflow transformation effort follow:

- Take full advantage of the IT system capabilities being provided by the vendor (achieve greater value from the investment made by the organization in the project).
- Reduce or streamline work processes through consolidation or elimination (reduce the cost of each unit of service delivered and improve staff productivity).
- Eliminate process gaps (opportunities for process failures or lost information).
- Improve the processes controlling handoffs between clinical and business teams.
- Improve team communication and staff satisfaction.

Today's imaging technologies generate massive amounts of data that must be used in generating a formal interpretation. Recent reports from the Society for Imaging Informatics in Medicine (SIIM; formerly the Society for Computer Applications in Radiology, or SCAR) suggest that as the complexity and volume of data increase, radiologists and other imaging professionals who do not have enhanced image processing, analysis, and viewing tools that transform the radiological interpretation process will be progressively challenged to maintain their performance and meet customer demands for information.[10] As data emerge from the ongoing work of this group, greater opportunities for workflow enhancement will become apparent and will likely drive IT system changes.

Referring Clinician Considerations

Most imaging IT systems are designed for use exclusively by radiology facilities, but PACS is the exception. PACS applications were originally designed exclusively for radiology use but have evolved over time to include general access applications for clinicians and specialty application tools that require special planning and close coordination with the referring clinician groups affected. The vendor project plans will include the technology deployment and setup for general Web access, but organizations will need to incorporate planning and coordination with the affected clinical groups.

Many organizations provide clinicians with general access to medical results as a part of their clinical information systems. For most of them, radiology reports are distributed using this mechanism. To reduce the cost of providing general access to images, the organization will need to plan for an interface of this system to the medical results system. If the organization is planning or implementing an EMR program, image access and the context in which it is provided will become increasingly important considerations for vendor selection and image access planning across the enterprise.

Community physicians who admit patients or refer patients to the organization will want access to results and images. The challenge is defining system access parameters and security policies to ensure patient confidentiality and access tracking under the Health Insurance Portability and Accountability Act of 1996 (HIPAA) regulations. The hospital will be responsible for ensuring compliance for anyone accessing the data. One way to address these concerns is to require that community physicians become users on the systems that they access. Although this mechanism will require them to be trained and to become familiar with these systems (instead of receiving e-mails with the results, for example), it makes HIPAA compliance easier to manage. Once broader electronic records are available and images and reports are included, community physicians will be able to quickly access a broad range of data about their patients that will make this training worth the investment and further enhance the organization's support for these key groups.

Some PACS physician users will require additional planning and clinician involvement in the system implementation. The implementation of image display capabilities in the operating rooms, intensive care units, and the emergency department will require careful coordination, development of specialty work lists, user interfaces, and in some cases specialty displays to meet the needs of physicians. Gaining their acceptance for these implementations will involve including these constituents early in the planning in order to design the system implementations to meet their clinical practice patterns and the physical space available.

Technical Aspects of Implementation

Integration Challenges

Some decisions about implementation are driven by the vendor's system design and must be decided late in the process. For example, organizations that have already implemented RIS and are beginning their PACS implementation will be able to consider their options for managing data flows through the new two-system combination. Recently, some PACS vendors have begun acquiring information systems capabilities, and information systems companies are partnering with PACS vendors to provide "integrated" solutions. Some believe that a merger of RIS and PACS will be the final outcome. The industry has experienced some merger and acquisition activity that would support this premise, although a real integration of systems and the supporting workflows have been slower to materialize. In the meantime, organizations should carefully evaluate and, when possible, implement tighter integration between RIS, PACS, dictation/speech recognition, clinical reporting, and using the Healthcare Enterprise (IHE) profiles. IHE, a collaborative effort between the Health Information Management Systems Society and the Radiological Society of North America, has developed a set of integration protocols that provide the framework for tighter integration between imaging IT systems and hospital clinical systems regardless of vendor.[11] Using these protocols takes advance planning and a good vendor relationship in which both parties commit to the work required to complete the integration. The result can be significantly improved workflow for radiologists and technologists with information readily available from a single device.

The second integration challenge is determining the RIS/PACS data flows for the user interface. Ideally, the radiology clinical staff will be able to view data from any radiology IT system. This is slightly different than accessing data from a single device, as it relies on tight systems integration to present data seamlessly between systems at a single device. Some RIS/PACS vendors offer RIS-driven workflow, which allows the RIS to manage the open work list, status tracking, and patient history across both systems. One immediate benefit of RIS-driven workflow is access to the complete patient history and reports even if the images are not available in the PACS. This capability could lead to greatly streamlined reading processes for radiologists who need to compare current examinations with previous studies still housed on hardcopy film. Another benefit is the capability to implement paperless workflow more readily, because most dictation/speech recognition systems are already interfaced to the RIS. To the extent that the PACS vendor of choice supports this workflow, the organization can achieve significant workflow benefits from designing toward a RIS-driven workflow method.

Storage

Most organizations are finding it necessary to explore or have implemented an enterprise data storage system. The goal of these systems is to enable ready access to information from multiple systems by all users, enable future data mining and data analysis, and reduce the overall cost and complexity of data storage.

Radiology IT systems, especially PACS, generate large amounts of data and storage costs for the enterprise to manage. As a result, data storage methods and the systems to be used need special consideration and planning. The storage solutions supported will no doubt affect the vendor-of-choice decision, especially if the organization has adopted a specific direction (such as storage area network) and has invested heavily in implementing that technology. Technical team members from the IT department should be actively involved in the delivery of the storage solution if this approach is adopted.

Once the organization determines that electronic records (such as patient history, reports, images, and billing records) are to be the primary data storage method, it must depend more heavily on the systems that electronically store the information. As a result, data redundancy (appropriate duplication of critical data in a secure server for use in the event of catastrophic loss of the main data source[s]) and system failover (automatic transition to the redundant system to provide continuity of operations) become critical to maintaining the integrity of, and access to, the electronic-only environment. Disaster recovery, once a luxury, has become an absolute necessity in the electronic records era.

The overall storage strategy for a multisite enterprise requires significant planning and data volume projections. Once these plans have been developed, a storage framework should be created to accommodate multiple years of storage for all the systems and constituents incorporated in the plan. Populating the storage framework with storage modules is best accomplished incrementally whenever possible, because the density of storage media continues to increase and the price has remained relatively stable—actually decreasing the cost of storage per megabit over time.

The vendor community has employed various storage technologies in system architectures for radiology. It is important to identify the data storage technology and ensure that it complies with institutional standards before completing the vendor selection.

HIS/EMR Integration

In the planning phase, the process and reasons for adopting a plan to conform to the EMR strategy were discussed. One outcome of this plan is the storage system decision mentioned in the previous section, but there are others. Clinical users of radiology IT data also need solutions to meet their clinical needs. In the past, for example, PACS vendors offered a solution for enterprise access that delivered Internet connectivity to the PACS. Adoption of electronic imaging has been varied, and many institutions must still deliver film and film-based services to many of their key customers. The Internet systems were designed with very general image-processing capabilities and limited tools to meet the clinical workflow requirements of clinicians. Surgeons report a need for surgical planning tools that have not been traditionally available, for example, and this need has forced many of them to continue to use film as their primary imaging interface.

Thus, the enterprise access model must be reconsidered to deliver something more clinically useful. The discussion of the planning phase suggested engaging key stakeholder clinicians to develop a list of system needs and requirements and eliminating data silos. Recall that data silos create barriers to access by imposing multiple systems with which the end user must interact. The vendor of choice should be capable of meeting the needs of the clinicians in the organization, or a plan for meeting those needs must be developed as a part of the project. The system that is successfully adopted by a large portion of the radiology referring physicians will most likely achieve the business value expected from the system.

Data Migration

As organizations make the transition to newer imaging IT systems, converting previously stored data will become critical to normal day-to-day operations within the department and across the enterprise. Organizations have realized that the data storage decisions they made with earlier procurements have made their data virtually inaccessible in the new system without a significant investment in data conversion. In some cases they are unable to convert some raw data into the newer formats. Data migration deserves serious consideration with any new procurement, whether to ensure standard data formats for the future or to convert data from older systems into the new. Organizations must plan for the cost, time, and potential access risk associated with these activities.

Training

The vendor will provide initial end-user training for the system. Some vendors offer training for all users of the system, and some prefer a train-the-trainer approach. The organization must take full advantage of the vendor's system training and design mechanisms to provide ongoing training for all users of the system. It is a good idea to involve institutional training in the design of the ongoing training program and to obtain training materials from the vendor if possible to ensure that staff is consistently trained in the use of the system.

Systems administrator training is typically more intensive and should begin immediately upon initiation of the vendor contract. Systems administrators should always be involved in the implementation project and, in some cases, will lead the implementation of the system. At go-live, the management of the system will complete the transition to the system's administrator team and IT staff.

System Operations and Maintenance

After the new IT system is operational for the first time, the real work of managing and maintaining the system begins. It is typical for the vendor to provide some level of maintenance of the system that includes the option to receive updates and upgrades to the software modules licensed by the organization. Although this feature will increase the cost of the service contract, it will allow the system to remain current without the need for additional capital planning for these modules. The amount of vendor-provided support the organization selects for other components of the system will depend on the internal IT expertise and staffing available to manage the hardware infrastructure, operating system, database, interfaces, and the like. Most vendors can provide end-to-end support should it be needed and will commit to service level agreements at any level of support.

Most imaging IT systems require some departmental support for data and system management. Some departments have full-time teams, and some coordinate support with IT staff members. The support model selected varies by site, the location of the system infrastructure, and the level of support provided by the department for day-to-day operations of the system (for example, data backup, help desk, table maintenance, and implementation of updates and upgrades).

Conclusion

Radiology will continue to face many challenges in delivering high-quality, timely services to its customers. The use of IT can enable the specialty not only to meet those challenges but also to improve the customer experience at the same time. Planning for, procuring, implementing, and maintaining IT is complex and requires experience with IT systems and the organizational will to do it correctly.

References

1. Shortliffe EH. Strategic action in health information technology: why the obvious has taken so long. *Health Aff.* 2005; 24(5): 1222–1233.

2. Ball MJ, Gold J. Banking on health: personal records and information exchange. *J Healthc Inf Manag.* 2006; 20(2): 71–83.

3. Frisse ME. State and community-based efforts to foster interoperability. *Health Aff.* 2005; 24(5): 1190–1196.

4. Gottlieb LK, Stone EM, Stone D, Dunbrack LA, Calladine J. Regulatory and policy barriers to effective clinical data exchange: lessons learned from MedsInfo-ED. *Health Aff.* 2005; 24(5): 1197–1204.

5. Hammond WE. The making and adoption of health data standards. *Health Aff.* 2005; 24(5): 1205–1213.

6. Huang HK. *PACS and Imaging Informatics: Basic Principles and Applications.* New York NY: Wiley; 2004.

7. SCAR Conference Reporter. Speech recognition technology finds a voice. Available at: http://www.diagnosticimaging.com/scarreport2002/speech.jhtml. Accessed May 7, 2007.

8. Brown CL, Howarth SP. The power of picture archiving and communication systems: strategic hospital considerations. *J Healthc Inf Manag.* 2004;18(4):19–26.

9. Haramati N. PACS and RIS: approaches to integration. *J Healthc Inf Manag.* 2000; 14: (3): 69–81.

10. Andriole KP, Morin RL. Transforming medical imaging: the first SCAR TRIP™ Subcommittee of the SCAR Research and Development Committee. *J Digit Imaging.* 2006;19(1): 6–16.

11. Integrating the healthcare enterprise technical framework. Available at: http://www.ihe.net/Technical_Framework/Index.cfm. Accessed June 10, 2006.

Chapter 14

Managing Digital Data

Mark A. Watts

> *Within imaging facilities, as in so many aspects of healthcare, technology is playing an increasing role in information and communications. The US government has sought to move this process along with standards governing the security of electronic patient health information and privacy of all patient information. To ensure compliant, secure, effective access to images and related patient information, the radiology administrator must work closely with IT professionals to build and manage an electronic data network that is reliable and that has built-in redundant systems and adequate capacity and storage for today and the near future.*

Mandated Electronic Data Security and Patient Privacy

One of the goals of HIPAA was to increase efficiency in the healthcare industry by promoting the use of standardized electronic transactions. Implementation of HIS, RIS, and PACS exemplifies this move toward electronic communications.

One of the many challenges inherent in the new technology, however, is the need to keep patient data secure and private at all times. To ensure that HIPAA provisions are implemented without compromising data security, the Centers for Medicare and Medicaid Services issued a set of security standards that apply to all electronic protected health information (see Box 14.1) and that must be complied with by healthcare providers that transmit health information electronically (including imaging centers and radiology departments within larger healthcare facilities). These standards, known as the Security Rule, are designed to ensure data confidentiality, integrity, and availability.

Security is an ongoing process; even facilities that have met initial compliance standards must continually monitor the effectiveness of their efforts, the need for additional staff training, and revisions made necessary by new technology. Radiology administrators who are managing the transition from paper and film to digital systems must incorporate the new Security Rule into the process. Careful documentation of many decisions related to the Security Rule is essential. There is considerable flexibility as to how compliance is achieved; for example, no specific technology is recommended.

Box 14.1 Protect More Than Patient Information

The Health Insurance Portability and Accountability Act (HIPAA) Security Rule applies to electronic patient health information. Other laws and sound business practice call for similar protection of other information. Therefore, when designing systems for HIPAA compliance, consider the full range of data commonly found on office electronic systems, including (but not limited to) the following:

- Patient health, demographic, and financial information.
- Physician and staff personal, employment, and financial information.
- Business records, such as financial records, practice patterns, quality assurance statistics, and strategic plans.
- Research and peer review information.
- Computer software, especially proprietary or customized software.
- Information about payors.

Facilities are encouraged to consider available resources, future technology plans, and constraints. Failure to comply with the HIPAA standards, however, can result in substantial fines and even imprisonment.

The Security Rule includes sets of standards, covering (1) administrative safeguards, (2) physical safeguards, and (3) technical safeguards, as well as (4) organizational policies and procedures, and documentation requirements. In the sections that follow, each standard is summarized. For full details and updates, go to www.cms.hhs.gov/HIPAAGenInfo/.

Administrative Safeguards

The administrative safeguards category is the largest. It has nine standards that require healthcare facilities to do the following:

- Implement policies and procedures to prevent, detect, contain, and correct security violations.
- Identify the individual who will be operationally responsible for compliance—a designated security officer.
- Implement policies and procedures that ensure that employees have appropriate access to electronic patient information—that is, that an employee can access the information, but only the necessary information, needed to do his or her job.
- Implement policies and procedures for authorizing access.
- Establish a security awareness and training program, including periodic retraining.
- Create policies and procedures to identify and report security incidents, including unauthorized access, use, disclosure, modification, and destruction of information.

- Develop a contingency plan to ensure the security of, and recover access to, information during and after an emergency that damages electronic information systems.
- Conduct ongoing, regularly scheduled evaluations of security policies, procedures, and systems to ensure continuing compliance.
- Obtain satisfactory assurances from vendors and other business associates that measures are in place to adequately safeguard shared patient information.

Complying with this set of standards forms the basis for the facility's security processes and is interrelated with the other three sets of standards. A key tool to achieving compliance is risk analysis and subsequent risk management. Risk analysis is the process of identifying potential security risks and determining the probability of each risk's occurring and the scope of its impact. Once these issues have been determined, risk management is the process by which a facility identifies security measures to reduce the risks to a reasonable and appropriate level, given financial, technological, and situational constraints. (The Centers for Medicare and Medicaid Services has developed a paper outlining the basics of risk analysis and management, which can be accessed at www.hipaadvisory.com/regs/FinalSecurity/index.htm.)

Physical Safeguards

The four standards governing physical safeguards aim to protect a facility's electronic information systems and equipment, and the buildings they are housed in, from natural or environmental hazards and unauthorized access. In applying these standards, the designated security officer and radiology administrator must consider not only office-based personal computers and modality equipment but also any devices that radiologists or other staff members may use to access patient health information. These devices include home personal computers, laptops, personal digital assistants (PDAs) and cell phones, especially those with text messaging and e-mail capabilities.

The physical safeguard standards require healthcare facilities to do the following:

- Implement policies and procedures that limit access while ensuring that properly authorized access is allowed. These measures should include access during an emergency, theft and tampering controls, building access control (for example, identification badges), and security maintenance documentation.
- Develop guidelines for proper use of workstations and other equipment on which patient information is created or stored.

- Devise a system to physically protect all workstations and related electronic devices from unauthorized users.
- Implement policies and procedures to ensure proper handling of hardware and all forms of electronic media (for example, optical disks, digital memory cards, and CD-ROMs) when they are being installed, moved, stored, or removed.

Most facilities will already have many of the necessary measures in place to comply with these standards, ranging from basic door and window alarms to inventory logs that track all equipment. However, documentation will be essential for compliance, especially with regard to storage media, which may be harder to maintain stewardship over than equipment with a more substantial physical presence.

Technical Safeguards

As mentioned earlier, all the standards are technology neutral and flexible to allow each facility to determine which security measures and technologies are reasonable and appropriate to achieve compliance. Thus, as with the other sets of standards, the technical standards present general directives, not technology proscriptions. These standards require healthcare facilities to do the following:

- Implement systems to provide users with access and the ability to perform functions on information systems, programs, or files, including a system to identify and track users, access information in emergencies, automate logging off, and encrypt data.
- Set up systems for audit controls and reports to track activity in patient information files.
- Implement procedures to protect electronic patient information from improper alteration or destruction.
- Set up a system to verify the identity of the person or organization seeking access to electronic patient information, such as using a password or personal identification number, a smart card, or a biometric (for example, a fingerprint).
- Implement technical security measures to protect electronic patient information as it is being transmitted by e-mail, Internet, the facility network, or other electronic means, including ensuring that the information is not improperly modified during transmission and encrypting information when appropriate.

More than any other set of standards, the technical safeguards call for close collaboration with the facility's IT staff. The National Institute of Standards and Technology (http://nist.gov) has created several publications to help IT staff analyze risk and achieve IT security.

Organization Requirements

The fourth set of safeguards addresses two areas relevant to imaging facilities. The first area is relationships with vendors and other business associates. For purposes of the standards, business associates may include other healthcare organizations, as well as general businesses such as software vendors or management consultants. The key factor is whether the business will have any access to electronic patient health information. If so, the standard requires a contract with the business associate that calls for the business to do the following:

- Implement safeguards to reasonably and appropriately protect all electronic patient information the business creates or has access to.
- Ensure that any subcontractors it uses agree to have safeguards in place.
- Report any security incidents to the imaging facility.
- Acknowledge that the contract may be terminated if the business fails to comply with the agreed-on security measures.

Compliance with this standard also requires the organization to take appropriate steps whenever it learns of a business's failure to comply with its security contract. These measures range from addressing the failure with the business to terminating the contract. (Radiology administrators working in Veterans Affairs facilities or other government healthcare facilities should review the full standard, as different specifications are established for compliance with this standard by government organizations.)

The second topic covered by the organization requirements that is relevant to radiology facilities is documentation. Specifically, organizations need to implement policies and procedures that are reasonable and appropriate, reflect the organization's mission and culture, and meet standards for sound business practices. The policies and procedures are to be

- Maintained in written form.
- Held for at least 6 years.
- Available to anyone responsible for carrying them out.
- Regularly reviewed and updated, as needed.

Patient Privacy

HIPAA addresses not only security as it relates to electronic patient health information but also the broader issue of patient privacy. The Privacy Rule took effect several years before the Security Rule, so most covered healthcare

SIDEBAR: Tips to Ensure a Smooth Road to Compliance

- Involve the most senior management in communicating the importance of compliance.
- Apply sanctions for compliance failure consistently and fairly to all employees and physicians.
- Provide adequate training, and repeat it as needed.
- Be aware that each staff member probably has his or her own view of what constitutes information confidentiality and security, and these views may need to be overcome before full compliance will be met.
- Consider that because access to information may equate to power, resistance to changes in access may be substantial.
- Acknowledge that a facility with a culture of openness—by choice or by necessity (as in the case of a small, freestanding facility)—may find resistance to security requirements such as mandatory logging off whenever a workstation is left vacant for even a short time. Employees may perceive such requirements as a sign that they are not trusted.
- Be prepared to deal with employee resistance to reporting compliance failures. Fear of retribution, lack of appreciation of the importance of reporting incidents, and hesitancy about "telling" on a co-worker are a few of the reasons employees fail to report. Take a lesson from the recent initiative to improve medical error reporting, and consider implementing a "no-blame" system that focuses on correcting reasons for noncompliance and not on punishing individuals who fail to comply.

organizations have measures in place to ensure compliance. Thus, the radiology administrator and the designated privacy officer (required by the rule) will primarily be concerned with ongoing compliance monitoring and retraining, when necessary. Because the Privacy Rule has standards related to ensuring privacy of patient information, some measures may achieve compliance for both rules.

As they relate to patient information, the two rules differ in two significant ways. First, the Privacy Rule, which is enforced by the US Department of Health and Human Services Office for Civil Rights (www.hhs.gov/ocr/hipaa), applies to all patient health information, including oral, written, and electronic information. The Security Rule addresses electronic information only and is enforced by the Centers for Medicare and Medicaid Services. Perhaps more significantly, the Security Rule provides substantially more comprehensive requirements and in greater detail to achieve compliance than does the Privacy Rule.

Under the Privacy Rule, patients have a right to expect that their health information will be kept private and confidential. Patients must be informed of their rights and of the measures they can take if those rights are abused. In particular, the standards call for the following:

- *Notice.* The patient should receive a "Notice of Information Practices" that outlines the patient's privacy rights and explains how his or her health information will be used and disclosed.
- *Access.* The patient has the right to see, copy, and supplement his or her own medical records. The health facility must provide a copy on request, but there may be a fee.
- *Security.* Any healthcare facility that collects, shares, and stores patient health information must have appropriate technical and administrative safeguards in place to protect that information.
- *Limits on disclosure to employers.* Healthcare providers cannot disclose a patient's identifiable health information to the patient's employer except in specific circumstances, such as a preemployment or postemployment physical examination.
- *Limits on disclosure to law enforcement.* In most cases, law enforcement officials must present some form of legal process (for example, a warrant, subpoena, or summons) before a healthcare facility can disclose a patient's health information to them.

The Privacy Rule also calls for healthcare facilities to take measures to inform patients of the actions they can take if they believe their rights and protections have been violated. These measures include the following:

- Contacting the facility's privacy officer to report the incident and seek resolution of the problem.
- Filing a complaint with the US Department of Health and Human Services Office for Civil Rights. This office has the authority to impose civil and criminal penalties if it finds a violation of the law.
- Seeking state-level recourse, especially if state privacy laws have also been violated. Among those likely to help are the state attorney general, insurance commissioner, and medical board (Box 14.2).
- Seeking legal redress in the state courts. Although a patient cannot sue a healthcare provider for a violation of the federal privacy law, a documented violation of the federal law may strengthen a privacy case brought in state court.

Box 14.2 Legal Regulations

Most states have laws and regulations governing patient privacy and health information security. However, when state law conflicts with the federal HIPAA rules, the federal rules apply.

Electronic Information Networks

A new patient arrives at the imaging facility, order in hand. In the 21st-century facility, patient care begins with the manual input of the patient's admission, discharge, and transfer information into the RIS. With the first keystroke on the computer, data with stored value are generated. If correctly transferred, protected, reviewed, and stored, these data are the basis for timely delivery of a clinically significant report and subsequent patient care decisions, as well as the justification for payment.

The registration workstation is connected to a network. The cornerstone of modern information systems is the data network. This statement is truer now than ever before because of the convergence of telephony, security, building controls, and storage within the data network. In IT, a network is a series of points, or nodes, interconnected by communication paths. Networks can interconnect with other networks and contain subnetworks. Without the network, few, if any, software applications would function.

When a facility's patient information system is based on film and paper, humans are responsible for transmitting, storing, and clarifying the data. However, a computer-based patient information system relies on electronic data transfer; for communication to occur among the various workstations and departments, some form of common language must be in place. Understanding the basics of communication protocols and integration can make selecting and managing the many elements of the electronic communications and interfacing modality devices easier and less prone to incompatibility issues.

Communication Protocols

Communication protocols, or standards, are specifications that allow software applications and electronic devices to exchange data without losing meaning (Figure 14.1). Devised by IT and content experts, often working through volunteer, not-for-profit organizations, the protocols are adopted as industry standards and are used by software developers, device manufacturers, and others in developing new products. Two common protocols within healthcare and radiology are HL7 and DICOM.

HL7—Health Level Seven is the organization that develops specifications governing applications to exchange key sets of clinical and administrative data, such as the RIS, but the protocols are commonly referred to as HL7. Physician orders, patient demographics, transcriptions, and billings are examples of data transferred with the HL7 protocol.

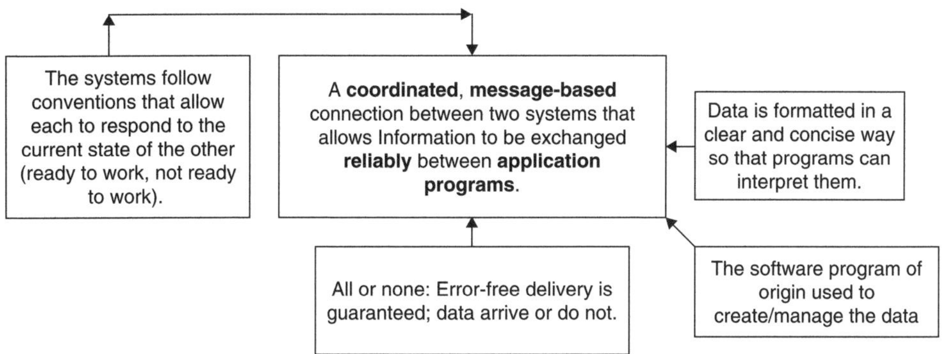

Figure 14.1 The key attributes of a communication protocol, such as HL7.

Before HL7, interfacing two healthcare applications involved a negotiation that had virtually no ground rules. Details as minor as record separators could be a source of disagreement and delay. Vendor preference, more than customer requirements, tended to influence the outcome. HL7 emerged as a response, providing a common vocabulary and architecture to tie the analysis/negotiation process much more closely to customer requirements. Whereas many other protocols focus on the needs of a specific department, HL7 focuses on the interface requirements of the entire healthcare organization.

Level 7 is the highest level of communications model established by the International Organization for Standardization. It supports software application functions such as security checks, user identification, availability checks, and data exchange structuring.

DICOM—The Digital Imaging and Communications in Medicine (DICOM) standard is used for the exchange of images and related information. It is DICOM that allows a computer to connect to a database, retrieve an image, or find out what images are stored in another part of the network. DICOM also can facilitate consistent image quality, media storage, security, information retrieval, and myriad other functions particularly relevant to settings, such as a radiology facility, in which a patient may have multiple scheduled procedures with multiple results.

All DICOM-compatible devices must provide a DICOM Conformance Statement. This statement describes the functionality of the device, such as which compression technology and media are supported. By reviewing this document before purchasing new equipment, the radiology administrator and IT staff can determine compatibility with existing equipment.

Another essential DICOM feature is the DICOM Modality Work List, which allows scheduling information to be retrieved by a modality. When the work list is installed, the technologist simply scans a barcode with the patient's unique identifier or selects the patient information from a menu, and the information is copied from the central HIS or RIS onto the screen. Information no longer needs to be manually reentered, significantly reducing the likelihood of errors. For example, one facility reduced data entry errors from 6.4% to 0.1%.[1]

The standard also includes a feature to achieve consistency in image presentation among various monitors. The DICOM Grayscale Standard Display Function specifies the luminance, so images sent from one device will appear the same on another, if both devices support the DICOM grayscale standard.

DICOM security mechanisms provide for encryption and electronic signatures when images and other kinds of patient health information are being retrieved by way of the Internet or other nonsecure modality. Another DICOM protocol standardizes exchange media so that images are stored in a standard format and can then be exchanged and read by another device. This protocol, for example, allows images produced by way of a portable ultrasonography unit to be stored on CD-ROM and then downloaded to a workstation.

The DICOM standard is continually updated and revised as needs are identified and technology changes. Only when revisions support new technology, however, will it be necessary to update other DICOM-compatible devices within the facility to ensure continuing interconnectivity.

Integrating the Health Enterprise

Developing information standards that govern computer functionality, such as HL7 and DICOM, is a crucial first step toward an effective EMR that will support the federal government's goal of building a national healthcare information network. But IT professionals and healthcare experts have recognized that the standards are not enough; a technical framework that describes workflow processes, identifies interoperability problems, and develops integration profiles to solve them is also needed. This goal is what the Integrating the Healthcare Enterprise (IHE) initiative is designed to accomplish.

Each year, IHE carries out a four-step process that results in better device connectivity and compatibility. First, clinicians and IT professionals identify common interoperability problems. Next, healthcare IT experts identify relevant existing standards and define how to apply them to the problem by issuing integration profiles. At the annual IHE Connectathon, vendors that have implemented the new profiles test their systems for interoperability, allowing them to resolve issues in a supervised testing environment. Finally, the vendors issue IHE integration statements that document the profiles their devices support. Radiology administrators and others who are issuing requests for proposals to purchase modality devices, computers, and other electronic equipment can reference the relevant integration profiles in the RFP, reducing the likelihood of incompatibility issues. For more information about IHE and its impact on the EMR, see www.ihe.net.

Electronic Network Reliability

As computer systems are increasingly integrated into the delivery of healthcare, their reliability becomes all the more critical. In the past, computerized systems in healthcare typically were limited to the HIS, RIS, billing systems, and other non-life-critical functions. But the recent industry-wide movement toward EMRs, PACS, and computerized bedside monitoring has increased the criticality of those information systems.

A panel discussion at an American Medical Informatics Association symposium in the late 1990s pondered the issue of system reliability. The panel commented that although 100% reliability may be desirable, it may not be affordable. Building highly reliable computer systems is expensive. Organizations need to make important resource allocation decisions that consider the risk to patients, the provider's time, the cost to the institution, and other factors.

Defining Reliability—Reliability must first be defined before it can be measured. Reliability can be measured from two perspectives: the clinician-centric perspective and the IT operational perspective. Both points of view are valid and necessary. The clinicians' perspective is concerned with the ability of clinicians to access one or more applications. A clinician's view is macroscopic: Does the application work? Can I access and record the information I need to treat my patients? Clinicians are concerned with the function of the complete application system—that is, the set of all components (for example, PCs, servers, disk drives, network devices, application software, and operating systems) that provide expected functionality to the user.

The IT staff members take the microscopic view. To increase reliability, the IT staff must identify which part of a system may be failing and then repair it. The IT staff must appreciate the complete application system while monitoring and repairing the atomic components of the system.

System Availability—The reliability of a system is commonly defined as the ratio of time the system is available during the time it is expected to be available. How does one define *acceptable downtime?* For example, for a system that is planned to be

Reliability Rate (%)	Actual Time Unavailable (hours)
99	87.6
99.50	43.8
99.75	21.9
99.90	8.8
99.95	4.4

continuously functional for 1 year, 99% reliability would mean that it would be down, on average, more than 87 hours annually. Clearly, this system may not be considered reliable (Table 14.1).

The cost of unreliable systems can be quantified by examining the cost of projected downtime. Estimate how many labor-hours would be lost during 1 hour of downtime during peak use. Multiply that number by the average salary of the people who could not do their jobs because of system unavailability. Add a factor for intangible costs, such as employee frustration, patient frustration, and patient safety. The resulting hourly figure can help justify using resources to strengthen reliability and selecting systems to accomplish that reliability.

Testing Reliability—Determining whether a system is functioning properly is not an insignificant activity. A system can never be completely, conclusively tested before deployment, and an application system cannot be 100% tested while it is deployed. Therefore, only a portion of system functionality may be examined to determine if the system is up and running properly. A system test may affect system performance temporarily, even if the effect is imperceptible. The radiology administrator and IT staff need to closely coordinate any planned test.

The optimal system test will be sentinel, minimally invasive, and timely. For a test to be sentinel, it must be truly indicative of application function. That is, if the sentinel test indicates that the application is down or up, it should genuinely be down or up. A minimally invasive test will have as little impact on the target (and other) systems as possible. Finally, if a test is timely, it will reveal problems as soon as they occur, helping maximize the IT department's ability to repair a problem before it is noticed, and minimize the downtime experienced by the users.

IT systems periodically require scheduled maintenance or upgrades that cause unavoidable downtime. Although controlled outages are preferable to unplanned downtime, they still affect clinical operations. The IT department should strive to minimize outages; it should also be encouraged to develop inventive and low-risk methods of maintaining systems while minimizing downtime.

Systems Management—An often overlooked, but essential, component of network management is the systems management hardware and software, also known as the *network management system.* This system alerts the organization when other systems degrade or fail. It also captures information about the use of scarce resources and can assist systems and network engineers and radiology administrators with IT trending, planning, and ultimately, budgeting.

The systems management strategy of a healthcare facility may be consolidated into a single system or be distributed among several off-the-shelf or homegrown applications. Either way, the technology is essential. Many strategies rely on redundancy to ensure reliability, but how useful is redundancy if there is no way to know when the primary system has failed and whether the secondary system has taken over? Redundancy without system management buys the facility one additional failure. Over time, that isn't likely to be enough.

System management software may also be used for anticipating problems before they occur and identifying trends in system activity and function. Assume, for example, that the use of available disk space is a constantly increasing function. Then assume a definable trend (for example, an increase of 50-mb per day, an increase of 5% per month, or a surge of disk space utilization on the last day of the month for reporting). If the trend is simple (that is, linear), basic regression analysis can tell the IT planner approximately when the current disk space will be fully utilized and when the facility should purchase additional disk space.

This sort of proactive monitoring ensures that the system will not be permitted to fail when resources are exhausted. It also provides for resources to be purchased "just in time." Considering that technology tomorrow is almost always less expensive than today, this strategy may reduce real costs.

Electronic Network Redundancy

Redundancy is the use of multiple components to fulfill the same function and is probably the most resource-intensive method of increasing system reliability. Redundancy may be used in several ways. In general, the more quickly and seamlessly the redundant system is integrated into the primary system, the greater the cost. Modern redundant systems may also be used simultaneously to increase performance so that the secondary system is not completely idle while the primary system is being used.

For servers and storage, documented and often-used methods can create redundant arrays of hard disks to ensure reliable storage. Through the use of a storage area network (SAN), a redundant array of inexpensive disks (RAID) can be configured between data centers miles apart. The costs increase with the sophistication of the solution, however. A host-based RAID can be reasonably inexpensive, whereas a completely redundant data center can significantly increase the overall IT expenditure. Each organization must decide how much insurance is enough.

Servers come in stateful and stateless redundancy. Stateful redundancy is the current state of the server; the applications running on the server, the processes, and associated data structures stored in random access memory can be transitioned to a new server with access to the same storage systems. Stateful redundancy has the advantage of being minimally disruptive. If done well, users may not even sense an outage. Stateful redundancy is rarely used, however, because it can be difficult to implement correctly.

Stateless redundancy is more common. Essentially, an active server and a passive server often connect to the same set of storage. When the active server fails, the passive server starts the processes formerly running on the active server. Then the passive server becomes the active server. This redundancy is often interruptive and requires users to restart their applications and reauthenticate.

The simplest forms of database redundancy employ RAID and passive server redundancy. These approaches protect the institution from disk failures but do not protect the data from errant database operations. If a database administrator types an inadvertent command, for example, neither of these methods offers protection. What is needed is a means of duplicating the data across multiple, independent disks and servers without allowing any "bad" transactions to be processed.

Database vendors and third-party vendors have built systems that stream transactions from a primary database to a secondary database. Whereas the primary database reflects a "live feed" of transactions, the secondary database reflects a time-delayed feed. This redundant system can be configured so that primary-to-secondary transactions flow in near real time, but the secondary system won't "play" the transactions until minutes or hours later to ensure that devastating transactions are not committed into the database.

In the event of a failure or data corruption of the primary server, the database administrator can instantly "play" the pending transactions on the secondary database server (except the last offending transaction) and promote the secondary server to the status of primary server.

Additional redundant systems introduce complexities that can challenge system management. For example, high-availability systems require communications between the redundant systems to ensure that both systems will not simultaneously attempt to become the primary system. Once again, the level of reliability and redundancy desired must be balanced against cost, complexity, and system management capabilities.

Data Recovery via Electronic Vaulting

Today's technology environment presents many options for data recovery, ranging from off-site tape storage to fully redundant off-site data mirrors, each of which has its own costs and benefits. An electronic vaulting solution is a viable alternative to off-site tape backups. Electronic vaulting drastically reduces a healthcare organization's recovery time and provides a cost-effective means for maintaining and achieving rapid restoration when compared with traditional tape-based recovery and online hot-replicated storage.

Electronic vaulting in the highly reliable infrastructure environment ensures the ability to restore from disk, which is significantly faster than conventional tape-based recoveries, at a cost below that of replicated hot storage. The electronic vault secures the transfer of data by using encryption over a dedicated line directly to the recovery facility, which meets HIPAA standards (see the earlier discussion) and avoids security and compliance risks inherently associated with the transportation of physical tapes to off-site locations. Electronic vaulting also sends compressed daily incremental changes, thereby lowering the bandwidth requirements over traditional replication solutions. An imaging facility may be able to eliminate some, if not all, of the traditional tape backup and off-site rotations, reducing the local backup costs of tape, management, and off-site storage.

The electronic vault uses multiple hard drives in a RAID. This technology compensates for the failure of an individual hard drive by writing the stored data across multiple drives. If one drive fails, the data are still intact.

Archiving and Storage Solutions for Digital Data

As more radiology facilities move from conventional film and paper media toward digital systems, and diagnostic imaging procedures produce ever larger image files, the strain on storage and archival systems becomes acute. Nuclear medicine, CT, MRI, and ultrasonography produce image files that range from 10- to 4,000-mb per procedure. The need for increased data storage is particularly acute in PACS technologies, which require storage for large volumes of data—as much as 1,000 times that of other healthcare applications.[2] As a result of this shift from plain-film radiography to more advanced imaging modalities, radiology administrators must have greater storage capacities and faster retrieval times.

Radiologic archives must meet several general requirements:

- The archives must be securely stored.
- Storage facilities must accommodate not only current data but also projected short-term capacity.
- The storage system must be able to store multiple, redundant, synchronized copies of the images and EMR to ensure HIPAA compliance.
- Media on which data are stored (for example, magnetic tape or disks) should have adequate capacity.
- An index or other mechanism must be provided to allow accessibility.
- Documentation must be provided to ensure compliance with HIPAA and other legal requirements for the chain of custody.
- The system should be easy to implement and operate.
- The archiving process must provide a mechanism for accurately and safely destroying outdated records according to HIPAA, legal, and facility policies and procedures.
- To protect the archives, the storage system should have an alerting mechanism (for example, e-mail notification) whenever a system failure occurs, a redundant power supply plugged into an uninterruptible power supply system, and an automatic data backup system.

Types of Storage—Three functional categories of storage are generally acknowledged: online, nearline, and offline. Offline storage is removable tape or optical media that are stored on a shelf and manually retrieved. It is slow and prone to error, so it is rarely used today.

Online storage, commonly used for active files, puts data on magnetic hard drives, which allows for access within milliseconds. Historically, hard drives were more expensive than other options, but that is no longer the case. Approximately 90% of studies that are in active use and stored in PACS are less than 1 year old, so experts recommend buying at least 1 year's worth of online storage capacity.[2]

Nearline storage historically incorporated a tape or optical "jukebox," which robotically retrieved the tape on which the needed data were stored and inserted it into a drive to read or write the data. Such a system accesses data within approximately 60 seconds. Radiology administrators who purchased early PACS usually stored most of their data on a nearline system because hard drives were costly. However, failure of the robotics, slow data retrieval, and substantial upfront costs made this alternative less than satisfactory.

At present, the preferred storage setup in many imaging facilities with PACS is online for active files and nearline for disaster recovery backup files and protection from online technological obsolescence. The nearline system is disk based, using hard drives rather than a jukebox.

Online Storage Configurations—Radiology administrators working in a PACS environment generally have had three configurations from which to choose when setting up online storage solutions. Direct-attached storage (DAS) involves having the storage hard drives directly on the PACS server. The main advantages are simplicity and relatively low cost. The system has two significant disadvantages, however. First, when the server goes down, access to all data is lost. Second, the system does not allow for significant expansion. A server is limited by the number of hard drives that can be fitted into it, so adding capacity is often difficult.

SAN is a second option. Storage is independent of the PACS servers because it is handled by a dedicated network that connects storage devices to computers. Storage can be accessed by more than one server, so stored data are available even when the server is not. SAN offers high performance and high redundancy, but it is more complex than DAS, is costly to install, and is specific to a given PACS software.

Finally, network-attached storage (NAS) is freestanding storage sitting on the network, not directly attached to the servers. It offers high performance, moderate pricing, and a good level of redundancy. Because NAS is not tied to the PACS software, the radiology administrator has greater flexibility in choosing the NAS vendor and system.

References

1. Yoshimura H, Inoue Y, Tanaka H, et al. Operating data and unsolved problems of the DICOM modality worklist: an indispensable tool in an electronic archiving environment. *Radiat Med.* 2003;21:68-73.

2. Nagy P, Farmer J. Demystifying data storage: archiving options for PACS. *Appl Radiol.* 2004; 33(5):18-22.

Chapter 15

Image Management

Ed Yoder

The film library is central to the mission of the medical imaging facility. By efficiently and accurately providing access to images, the staff members make an important contribution to quality patient care. Film libraries, like other areas of healthcare, are in transition in many facilities as they face a move from analog, film-based files to electronic systems. Nevertheless, the functions of a film library remain much the same: to manage, archive, inventory, access, loan, retrieve, and process thousands of images. Radiology administrators face the challenge of physically organizing the library; staffing it with motivated, trained individuals; and establishing procedures to ensure that these functions are performed promptly, accurately, and efficiently.

From the discovery of the x-ray to today, the management of radiographic and other medical images has been a continuing source of frustration for healthcare facility managers. The film library is at the heart of the traditional analog medical imaging facility, where the functional processes needed to manage, archive, inventory, access, loan, retrieve, and process the medical information contained in every imaging file occur on a continuous basis. In the 21st-century electronic facility, the processes are automated and some of the terminology has changed, but the functions remain the same. Image retrieval for comparative review—also referred to as *fetching* and *pre-fetching*—continues to be the core function of the film library in both analog and electronic configurations.

In the analog facility, when someone needs to locate an image, he or she looks to the film library. As such, it is imperative that the film library use a consistent, concise filing system so that film records can be located quickly and efficiently. The process is essentially similar to that of a public library, the purpose of which is to house, inventory, loan, retrieve, and provide custodial care for books belonging to the community. When a patron desires to obtain a book to read, the library staff retrieves the book and makes it available for checkout. When the patron fails to return the book at the appointed time, the library staff must proactively respond by reminding the patron of the responsibility to return the book for others to use. Similarly, the film library is the central repository of image files, and its staff must perform the same functions as any other type of library to ensure that use of the image files is maximized for each consumer.

Without an effectively managed film library, the movement of images for interpretation becomes inefficient. Whether the library system is analog or electronic, the needs of its consumers remain the same, and the effects of ineffective access to images on the rest of the medical community are significant.

The Physical Setting of the Analog Film Library

The film library is a place where physicians congregate, so it should remain clean, organized, and professional at all times. An area within the film library itself should be available where physicians can comfortably review images to decrease the likelihood of image loss. (Of course, images and reports can still disappear from the physician work area, because physicians may leave with the images they are reviewing.) The design of the film library viewing area should enhance the referring physician's workflow. The space should be easy to use and be located in an area that will stimulate physician use and efficiency. Such a space will decrease the likelihood that physicians will request that images, read and unread, be delivered to other areas within the hospital, to a clinic, or to another working location.

Within the film library itself, the work areas should be designed for efficiency, with counters at standing and sitting heights. A work area that is appropriately designed with good lighting, air return and cooling, and appropriately placed equipment will enhance employee productivity and promote good employee morale. Providing employees with the tools they need to do their jobs will enhance their ability to perform good work that is error-free.

Organization of the Electronic Film Library

Many of the functions and much of the organization of an analog film library also apply to the effective operation of an electronic film library. Access to images by the local medical community is still critical. Although physicians may no longer physically go to the film library to review an image, they still require access to the images. It is still necessary for someone to manage image flow to ensure that all images for a particular imaging study are contained in the patient's image file and that electronic misfiling does not occur.

The physical organization of the film library in an electronic environment is no less important than in an analog environment. Even though the actual film library may be smaller than in the traditional analog environment, work spaces and work surfaces must still be ergonomically configured with the appropriate lighting, heating, and cooling. Proper staff training (to be discussed later) is even more crucial, as the staff in the electronic environment will be providing continuous training to physicians, nurses, and other paramedical personnel in the access and retrieval of images, as well as in the use of the many image manipulation functions inherent in the PACS environment. Users will always ask basic questions such as "How do I get to these images?" and "Has Mr. So-and-So's imaging study been performed and read?"

Basics of Image Tracking

Film library operations, in both analog and electronic environments, must be well organized. If they are not, the result will be lost film records in the analog environment and lost (orphan) images in the electronic environment. These losses can be particularly annoying for referring physicians who are unable to get images or reports from the film library. Once referring physicians become frustrated, it is hard to win back their confidence.

Film libraries traditionally have been organized with shelving units and terminal filing by medical record number or some other unique identifier; they have been staffed around the clock. Historically, the management of images in and out of the film library was accomplished using a card file; a staff employee would note the use of the film record on a card with the date, time, and borrower. More recently, the development of the RIS has enabled many healthcare facilities to replace the manual card file with electronic file tracking. In either system, the tracking of images and reports in and out of the film library is essential.

Many vendors offer image management software programs, which are usually part of the RIS. Many of these applications use a barcode, which improves efficiency, streamlines the management of image flow, and improves staff effectiveness. However, these advantages come with a cost. RIS packages and independent record-tracking systems add costs in software and hardware maintenance, repairs, upgrades, and replacements.

Computerization of film library functions, however, enables the facility to track images from the library to the radiologist and then back; from the library to the patient or referring physician as a loan; or from the library to various hospital nursing floors, intensive care units, and operating rooms. This ability to track image record use is a great resource. When a borrowed image jacket is tracked, not only is it better managed; also, the borrowing party can be held responsible for its return. Images and image jackets are commonly found in the trunk of a physician's car, tucked away in the darkest corner of the operating room, or on a shelf in the referring physician's office closet. The physicians involved may believe the image has been returned or claim ignorance of how the image came to be in an unauthorized location. Hospitals that have medical students and medical residency programs are at an increased risk for lost images, because medical education programs often remove image files from general access to use them for case study review with the senior medical staff. In any case, the images must be available for review. A reliable tracking system will provide some credibility so that film record borrowers can be held accountable.

The RIS also might have the capability to generate letters when loaned images are past due. Regardless of the capabilities of the system, each healthcare organization should develop policies and procedures for image record borrowing that dictate the length of time an image is allowed to remain away from the facility and follow-up actions that will occur when the images are not returned in the expected timeframe.

In particular, no one referring physician should be allowed to have a substantial number of film records on loan for an extended period. These film records are not available for use by other referring physicians or for use in comparison with new image studies. In addition, the absence of images from the film library creates inefficiency in the utilization of staff resources because of extraordinary amounts of time spent on the telephone tracking down missing image file jackets. Timely and repeated follow-up will decrease the likelihood that images will accumulate in a referring physician's office.

Analog Film Library Operations

In most healthcare facilities, images, image records, image files, and related medical information move 24 hours a day, 7 days a week. As such, certain processes need to be followed to ensure that the images and image files arrive on schedule to their various destinations. The film library responsibilities include the following:

- Processing new images.
- Retrieving images.
- Filing interpreted (read) images and filing previously borrowed images back into the system.
- Loaning out patient images.
- Ensuring clinical access to images.

In an analog facility, the film library must also ensure that all images are displayed for the radiologist to read daily and that comparison images are available as needed.

Hospital-based film library staff members must also ensure that images that need to go to nursing floors and patient rooms (for example, medical/surgical units, orthopedic units, coronary care units, intensive care units, operating rooms, the emergency room, and postanesthesia recovery units) arrive in a timely fashion to meet the needs of the attending physicians, hospital staff, and patients themselves.

Managing New Files

Facilities use any of several variations of a process for managing new images when they are produced. The basic procedure calls for the film library staff to prepare a new image jacket or modify an existing jacket with appropriate patient information and details of the radiologic examination being performed. This image jacket is then collated with the new images and transported to the radiologist for interpretation. This process can be completed by the technologist, film library staff member, technical aide, or supervisory staff member. When the radiologist has interpreted the image, it is placed in a file or bin and transported back to the film library, where the image is matched with the report and then filed within the film management system.

Images transported to the radiologist viewing area may be managed using several different methods. In settings where the radiologist uses a flat or angled viewbox, the images may be left in a stack for the radiologist. In settings where a multiviewer (such as a rotator or alternator) is used, the staff hangs the images on the multiviewer, often recording the space and frames used to hang these images on a log sheet. The location of these images is tracked in the computer system using predefined designation descriptions. It is the film library staff's responsibility to check the patient's image jacket for any previous images that may be needed for image interpretation. If a computerized information system is available, doing so is simple. If a patient has had previous images made and has visited the imaging facility on one or more occasions in the past, the jacket will reflect these visits and contain the previous images. The previous images are then hung next to the new images. Each radiologist will specify his or her preferred hanging sequences, and film library staff members should accommodate these preferences to allow the radiologist to be more productive and read faster.

Effective image management will track the location of new and previous images to the radiologist reading area and back, once report dictation is complete. The completed jacket should then go into a separate area within the film library, where it is checked for completeness and accuracy. Each jacket that is returned from the radiologist reading area should be checked before filing to reduce the occurrence of lost or misplaced images. The jacket then waits in this area for the report to be transcribed. Staff members file the completed report in the image jacket, which is then filed in the film archive.

Managing Image Retrieval

Retrieving and delivering images to various departments within a healthcare facility as requested are also critical film library functions. In general, set times are scheduled, during the operational hours of the library, when a staff member will make image and image jacket deliveries. During these scheduled stops, images are delivered as requested, and images that are ready for return can be picked up for re-filing in the film management system. Images ready for return should be left in a designated area so the film library staff will not erroneously take an image that is still needed for review. In large facilities, the library commonly establishes reading areas within the units, where images can be reviewed. This system supports a decentralized film management philosophy but requires more training of clinicians and more management oversight of the satellite locations. Lost images are still a real possibility and cannot be entirely eliminated.

Timely and accurate filing of interpreted images and previously borrowed image jackets back into the film management system is crucial. Images ready for filing should be sequestered in a separate designated area so they are not confused with outgoing images or images being readied for interpretation by the radiologists. Organization is again the key. Staff members assigned to this task must be detail oriented. They should understand the terminal digit filing system (or whatever system is being used) and how numbers are filed in chronological order. These staff members should be able to spot misfiled images and be alert when filing image jackets into the system. These employees need to be fast, but accurate; misfiling can result in many lost labor-hours in image retrieval.

An effective filing system also establishes appropriate clinical access to the organization's images. One of the more important functions of the film library is to maintain this access. Physicians must be able to view patient images at any time. Often these images are decisive factors in a patient's treatment. When images are not readily available because of poor filing systems, incompetent filing staff, image loss, misfiling, theft, and late returns, physicians will become frustrated and lose faith in the film management system. Patient care may suffer. An organized method for managing image files with an appropriately trained staff that understands the consequences of misfiled image jackets and lost images will reduce physician frustration and compromised patient care.

Managers must ensure that film library staff members take pride in their job responsibilities. Teamwork with the other units of the imaging facility is essential to integrate the film library staff into the entire image facility film management process. Pride, teamwork, and an understanding of job importance, along with error reduction strategies, are fundamental to managing a well-organized film library. Departmental quality initiatives can focus on eliminating filing errors, with success in achieving low error rates a reason for celebration throughout the entire facility.

Managing Patient Access to Records

Patients will need to take their film and digital images to other healthcare providers for review. Patients generally feel no obligation to return the images to the film library, although it is in their best interest to do so. They are not bound by film library policy, so often the only recourse is repetitive phone calls to obtain the files' return. Unfortunately, patients are not the only borrowers who may be cavalier about returning images. Other healthcare organizations may not share the film library's philosophy of properly managing images in their possession that do not belong to them. Therefore, despite the cost, most film libraries use copies, rather than original images, in their loan programs.

Many organizations send out only copies of the original images. An exception is made when a court order requires an original, in which case a copy is retained in the facility with the original file jacket in case the original images are not returned. Another noted exception occurs when federal, state, or local legislation or regulations require release of an original image for a predefined purpose. For example, ACR accreditation guidelines for mammography require that an original mammographic image be released to the patient on request for follow-up care at any other facility. Again, a copy, along with the original file jacket, should be retained within the film library.

Film library personnel must deal with HIPAA issues daily, and understanding these rules and regulations is important. The film library staff must follow this law; conformance must be 100%. Violating HIPAA regulations can result in fines and even prison time for serious violations.

The release of medical images and image files (whether electronic or film based) must comply with HIPAA guidelines. Anyone involved in the continuing care of a patient has "a need to know" and can request image and medical record information on that patient. However, before loaning images or image file jackets to patients, film library staff members are required to obtain two sources of identification from patients to ensure they are who they say they are. If patients do not have the appropriate identification with them, they may be upset and unable or unwilling to return. If this happens, facility protocols must specify what should happen next. Calling the medical records department and having the patient verify birth date and Social Security number will meet the identification requirements without inconveniencing the patient. If organizational policies dictate how to handle such situations, staff members will be well prepared when the need arises. Having clear and concise policies and thorough training can avoid staff confusion and mistakes.

Managing Archiving and Storage

Image archival systems (both film and electronic) are heavily space dependent. In the traditional film archive, large areas are usually arranged with stacks and rows of shelves. Because physical floor space is a vital commodity for most healthcare facilities, radiology administrators may find themselves challenged over the allocation of premium space for a function that does not generate any cash flow. However, the image archive is essential if the imaging facility is to maintain any reasonable level of quality in patient care.

Medical images must not only be managed so current images can be reviewed for patient care; they also must be retained for future patient care. The actual time necessary for image retention is determined by federal and state laws and regulations, so actual retention criteria differ from state to state. Pediatric images, mammography images, workers' compensation images, and asbestos exposure images often must be retained longer than general images, so the manager of an image archive must understand the specific requirements and laws governing the facility.

Because space is often limited in healthcare organizations, many facilities are forced to divide the space needed for retaining images into two or more categories—usually short-term storage and long-term storage. Short-term storage is considered to be an area that holds 1 to 2 years of image jackets. This area is usually within the imaging department or within close proximity. If space is limited, this area may not be located near the imaging department but will still be located somewhere within the facility. Some organizations even have a short-term file area that resides within the actual film library. This area holds 1 to 3 months' worth of image file jackets, the most commonly requested files.

If space is severely limited, the film library may not be able to store 1 to 2 years of images on site. Instead, it may be forced to retain a 2- to 3-month archive on site and store all other files off site. These storage facilities may be owned and staffed by the imaging department or its affiliated health facility. Alternatively, a vendor may be used to store images off site. When a vendor is used for off-site storage, a fee is charged for each image jacket archived, and commonly another fee is charged each time a jacket is pulled, regardless of the reason.

Either of these storage solutions or any variation of them is considered long-term storage. Generally, however, the term *long-term storage* covers inactive jackets with images that are 2 to 3 years old and older, depending on the state laws for retaining images.

Facilities with short- and long-term storage incorporate the moving or purging of image jackets into routine tasks. As images reach the predetermined maturing age, they are moved to the next archive level. For example, an organization might have a 3-month file located within the film library; an additional 2 years of storage on site within the film library; and another 5 to 10 years of storage (as dictated by local, state, or federal regulations) at an off-site facility owned or leased by the organization or provided as a service from an entity that manages records on a professional basis. When an image jacket in the 3-month file ages to 4 months old, it is moved to the 2-year storage. As the 2-year file area fills, jacket contents must be condensed to make room for the new jackets from the 3-month file. Additional room is created each year in the 2-year file as the second year of image jackets ages. When these jackets reach the 3-year maturity level, they are moved to long-term storage off site. To create room within the long-term storage, image jackets that reach the maturity level at which they are no longer required by law to be retained are pulled from the file shelving and discarded. Film file staff must follow HIPAA mandates for appropriate disposal of images and corresponding reports and patient information. A partnership with a vendor that shreds and discards sensitive information is recommended, and HIPAA partnership agreements must be signed.

Electronic Film Library Operations

In an electronic environment (PACS), it is still necessary to manage new image production, collate new images with historical images, and provide image access to the medical community on demand. Although some of these functions are automated, the oversight of the system and the management of the services must still be orchestrated by human activity. In some facilities, some of these functions have been assigned to members of the technologist staff, but in other facilities members of the traditional film library staff have been retrained to manage the PACS activities. Many combinations of staffing are used to manage the electronic imaging environment; the best combination depends on individual facility need, resource availability, cost, and management philosophy.

Managing Files

In the electronic film library, electronic patient folders must be created, and the new image must be placed electronically into the new folder. Although this filing is performed automatically by some PACS systems, human oversight is necessary to ensure quality control of patient images. Patient information and demographics must be correct and match those on the new image. Once the image has been interpreted, a staff member must make sure the correct report matches the new image. The report and image are then filed in the electronic image archive, which can be retrieved by anyone, anywhere, as long as that individual has been granted privileges to view the images within the PACS. Broken studies, orphan images, images that do not match patient information and demographics, missing images, images marked incorrectly, or incomplete imaging studies must be managed by staff members. Often the PACS administrator, or the PACS administration team in larger facilities, will fix or assign someone to fix these problems, which present themselves daily in an electronic environment. In many facilities, film library staff members can be trained to help solve these issues when they occur within the system.

Theoretically, in an electronic environment, the image is always available for review, and lost images become a thing of the past—at least that is the promise of PACS. However, this is not always the case. As with any electronic system, hardware failure and software glitches create situations in which an image is not available when it is needed. These situations require human intervention. Staff members must be trained to address physician frustration and needs during times when electronic images are not available.

Filing errors and lost images are for the most part eliminated in the PACS environment, although disruptions in network communications can create orphan images in the stream of data. The need for image management is still present, as files must be matched to the correct folder and images must be distributed electronically and by way of multimedia formats (CDs and DVDs). Physicians, nurses, and other healthcare staff members periodically need help with image retrieval in a PACS environment, and film library staff members can take on these tasks, especially during slow times.

In an electronic film library, the need to hang new images along with the corresponding comparison images still exists, but doing so does not generally require human intervention. Radiologists will develop hanging sequences or protocols in tandem with the PACS administrator; all images received within the PACS system—both new and previous—will automatically be loaded in the established sequence for the radiologist. However, a staff member must manage the patient files and ensure that all electronic images are located within the correct files. Someone must electronically validate the completeness of the imaging study before the radiologist opens it for reading, just as is done in a film-based environment. In many PACS configurations, images obtained after the image file has been opened for reading cannot be placed into that same examination file. These images are "orphaned" by the system and must be manually placed into the right file. Because of this situation, radiologists sometimes must reread a study because of an incomplete file.

Managing Patient Access to Records

The conversion from film-based imaging to electronic imaging does not change patients' needs for access to their image files. Many radiology facilities are using CDs to provide images to patients who need to carry them to another physician for further consultation. With the development of 64-slice CT scanners, however, the volume of data for each image file has increased significantly, so a single CD cannot accommodate the entire patient image file. In these cases, facilities are using multiple CDs or a DVD, which holds more data than does a CD. The problem is that not all physicians' offices have the electronic capability to view DVD images. Nevertheless, in the electronic environment, the original image continues to reside in the archive, and an exact copy is provided to the patient on a transferable medium. No resolution is lost, as is the case with copy film, and the medium for the copy is less expensive than copy film.

Managing Disaster Recovery

Film images are not indestructible and are susceptible to fire and water damage. An analog film library takes whatever measures are necessary to eliminate, as much as possible, these risks and to preserve the film-based image file. Once film is gone or damaged, it is irreplaceable. Historically, healthcare facilities have not been expected to maintain a duplicate or redundant film archive.

In a PACS environment, however, the media for maintaining an electronic archive provide an opportunity to duplicate images fairly easily and with minimal labor resources. Storage is more easily expanded than in the film environment and often does not require a significant increase in floor space.

Whereas film media have undergone regular cost increases, exclusive of industry changes in discount structure, electronic storage media have decreased in cost exponentially over time. As an example, an electronic archive of image files in 1999 could be placed on magnetic optical disks with a 1-terabyte archive for a cost between $700,000 and $1,000,000. In 2006, a 20-terabyte drive for a storage area network device or a network area storage device could be purchased for $120,000.

For these reasons, the expectations for electronic archives have gone beyond the traditional expectations for film archives; full redundancy is now expected. Full redundancy is not the same as having a system backup, which is a copy of the database. True redundancy includes having duplicate servers and duplicate archives. Redundancy provides for disaster recovery, whereas backup does not.

In a redundant configuration, the PACS archive is duplicated, often at an off-site facility miles away from the organization—even in another state. Vendors also offer a redundant solution, again usually in a different state than that of the client. (Chapter 12 further explaines the PACS environment and its associated storage systems and redundancy plans.)

SIDEBAR: Film File Room Operations

Film file rooms are still common in facilities across the United States, although many facilities have switched to a filmless environment. Some of the same issues and challenges exist in an electronic environment as in a film environment. The issues do not vanish with film; they just change format. Issues related to both environments include the following:

- The physician setting.
- The organization of the image library.
- The basics of image tracking.
- Library operations.
- The creation and management of new files.
- Management of image retrieval.
- Management of access to records.
- Management of archive and storage issues.
- Management of disaster recovery.
- Human resources and staffing.
- Recruitment.
- Employee retention.

Human Resources and Staffing

Recruitment and retention of qualified staff are two important, challenging issues that a radiology administrator faces when trying to staff a film library department. Although the library performs one of the most important functions of a medical imaging facility's operation, its staff is paid the least. Because of this fact, finding qualified candidates can be challenging; most applicants will have had little, if any, experience in a medical imaging film library environment.

Maintaining a film library filing system is a crucial part of imaging operations, yet the industry has not placed much emphasis on the value of attracting highly

---

qualified employees to this field. With the transition to an electronic archive with PACS, it will be unfortunate if the radiology community neglects to address this issue and continues to leave the management of the patient image files in the hands of the lowest-paid members of the staff.

Staff Recruitment

In most facilities, recruiting individuals to fill vacant positions within the film library should involve the human resources department. Hiring individuals with certain skill sets is key in this recruitment process. The film library requires individuals who pay attention to details. Having a solid understanding of terminal digit filing systems and chronological numbering are essential skills for employees, as is the ability to identify out-of-sequence numbering and other details such as name spelling and numerical coding. Prospective candidates for these positions usually will not have demonstrated these skill sets in previous jobs, because these candidates come from all walks of life. Therefore, it is essential that human resource professionals develop or implement testing measures to identify these skill sets in candidates.

Communication skills should also be evaluated, as library staff members often create the first impression a physician has of the facility as a whole. Film library staff should be friendly and willing to help, with a positive attitude; applicants should be able to handle individuals with difficult personalities while remaining polite and helpful.

Taking the time to find the appropriate candidates and create a pool of candidates from whom to select will significantly reduce error rates and misfiling within the film library. It is better to leave a position vacant and cover the vacancy with over-time staff than to hire the wrong person. Hiring the right person for the job should be the first priority.

Once a candidate has cleared human resources screening, he or she is ready to interview within the imaging facility. If preliminary screening is done by the human resources department, the radiology administrator will be interviewing only candidates who have been predetermined to be qualified for the job.

The face-to-face interview is one of the most important tools in the selection of prospective candidates. The interview's main purpose is to match candidates to the jobs for which they are applying and to fit them into the workplace. The interview is an opportunity to tell candidates what job functions are expected of them, what the imaging facility is like, and what the organization overall is like. It is not a time to sugar-coat the facility or the job and its requirements. Turnover within the first month of a new job generally results from the new employee's ill-informed expectations.

The interview is an opportunity to match the candidate's qualifications, work habits, personality, and attitude with those of the imaging department and the entire organization. Some facilities use employee (peer) interviews as well, allowing current employees to interview prospective candidates. Studies have shown that if employees are involved in choosing their new team members, they become more vested in the new employees' orientation and training.[1]

Employee Retention

Retention of current employees is another important aspect of human resources that should be a top priority for radiology administrators. Keeping employees happy and feeling that they work at a great place is extremely important. Retention is a complex concept and requires involvement by both human resources and management staff. Commonly, retention programs are implemented organization-wide rather than within an individual department.

Levering and Moskowitz[2] have studied workplaces to identify key characteristics cited by employees as making them feel they work for great places. In their book *The 100 Best Companies to Work for in America*, the authors explore these key areas:

- Employee participation.
- Sensitivity to the problems and issues of working mothers and fathers.
- More sharing of the wealth.
- Fun in the workplace.
- More trust between management and employees.

Listening to employees is probably the single most important tool a radiology administrator can use. In an open atmosphere, employees will say what they need; if the manager listens, the facility will retain the employees. If they feel unappreciated or not valued, they will leave. In addition, Studer argues that the key to "hardwiring the healthcare flywheel" to achieve excellence is providing the tools staff members need to do their jobs and a work environment that has a worthwhile purpose and meaning.[1]

Retention of energetic and skilled employees at the lower end of the pay scale also presents a challenge, because as they continue to excel they are often lured away by higher-paying jobs within or beyond the organization. Constant recruitment, orientation, and training can wear on the available resources and cause additional overtime as current staff members scramble to cover vacant shifts. Therefore, employees must be made to feel a vital part of the medical imaging team and be rewarded for excellence in the work they perform. The employees should feel rewarded and recognized when they perform duties that go beyond what is expected. Motivation and purposeful, worthwhile work are what all employees expect in a workplace, and the film library (analog or electronic) is no exception.

One factor that can affect staffing and retention within the film library is the transition to an electronic imaging environment. Initial discussions about a PACS program will cause unrest among employees because of fear of job loss. However, the transition to an electronic PACS environment does not eliminate the traditional film library, but instead replaces former job tasks with new electronic job tasks. Fear of job loss can be addressed by showing how PACS will actually result in the creation of new job opportunities for traditional film library employees.

In an electronic environment, film handling is obsolete. The image file jacket becomes an electronic file transferred over a network infrastructure to computers and computer workstations throughout the facility. The adoption of PACS will at least temporarily disrupt the work life of film library personnel; new job functions are created, and many existing job functions are in flux as they are transitioned to an electronic environment. Someone still has to make sure that image files are complete before being sent to radiologists for reading. Someone still must provide support to physicians and others in accessing images for their use. Someone still must provide image files in a transportable medium for patients who desire medical consultation at another healthcare facility. The challenge is to retrain support staff, who were not originally hired to perform computer-based functions. Some will be able to adapt to the transition, whereas others will not.

In an electronic environment, a PACS administrator is needed to run and manage the system. The administrator will require support staff to help him or her orient and train physicians, nurses, and various other staff members on how best to use the system. Staff will be needed to manage the upkeep of the system and handle the problems associated with the new environment, such as managing broken studies and patient electronic image folders. Many members of the traditional film library staff can be trained to be assets in a PACS environment, often becoming "super-users" who help others when they run into problems with the system.

Managing the fears of the film library staff about losing their jobs is important, as it will help determine the morale of the facility during this transition. Having discussion groups and involving the film library personnel in the change process will be key to alleviating their fears. Having members of senior administration outline how they expect the job changes to occur also will be important. If job eliminations are necessary, most organizations encourage attrition to achieve cuts—that is, not replacing an individual who leaves or relocating employees to other departments with open positions that match the employees' skills. In the transition to a PACS environment, process changes, job function redefinition, and job elimination generally can be planned, staged, and managed over time.

Determining staffing levels in either the traditional film library or the electronic PACS environment can be challenging. Film library staff members do not produce workload volumes in terms of procedures or relative value units. Thus, these employees do not generate revenue, but they provide critical support functions within the imaging facility that enable individuals who do generate revenues to be successful. Multiple resources are available to benchmark staffing levels and to support changes in those staffing levels. Some of these resources are listed on the AHRA Web site (www.ahraonline.org).

Conclusion

The film library in both the traditional film environment and the electronic PACS environment is the heart of the imaging facility. Ineffective recruitment, staffing, retention, and training all lead to disruptions in service. Ineffective protocols, processes, and procedures also disrupt service to the point of bringing patient care to a near standstill. Therefore, the overall management of the film library is as important in the day-to-day operation of the imaging facility as any other management function or activity. Without an effectively managed film library and image management program, the imaging "product" will not be delivered to the end consumer, the referring physicians.

In the future, the way many of the tasks and functions associated with the traditional film library are carried out will change. PACS will replace the analog film library and bring with it new twists on old problems, such as archiving, storage space, and disaster recovery. Yet some film-based tasks will remain in a manual format, and the tasks that are converted to electronic functions will need human oversight.

Qualified individuals will be needed to help manage the electronic system. Some of the film library staff will be trained in new computerized functions, and some will move elsewhere. Communication during transition, as always, is essential to provide an environment in which information goes both ways between staff and management.

Whether analog or electronic, the film library depends on recruitment and retention of employees with the appropriate skill sets to meet the expectations of the organization and its physicians. Good interviewing skills and accurate job expectations for the prospective candidate will help ensure that the right person is hired.

The transition to an electronic imaging environment through the acquisition and installation of PACS will provide solutions to many of the traditional problems associated with a film-based environment, but this change will also bring with it many new challenges. Overcoming obstacles such as staffing issues, patient record access, electronic conversion dilemmas, archive redundancy, and disaster recovery, in addition to the many process challenges associated with implementing and operating an electronic system for image management, is time-consuming. Nevertheless, the film library's contribution to the radiology facility's mission makes the effort worthwhile.

References

1. Studer Q. *Hardwiring Excellence: Purpose, Worthwhile Work, Making a Difference.* Gulf Breeze, FL: Fire Starter Publishing; 2003.

2. Levering R, Moskowitz M. *The 100 Best Companies to Work for in America.* 2nd ed. New York, NY: Penguin Group; 1993.

Chapter 16

Organization Files

David Fox and Patti Hoehn

Records exist for the information they contain. Maintaining an organization's records in a safe, secure, and orderly manner ensures that the information will be available when it is needed and be available to the appropriate individuals. Effective records management includes systematic creation, maintenance, and disposition of both paper and electronic files.

Being organized is not just a state of mind. As organizational specialist Julie Morgenstern has written, "Organizing is the process by which we create environments that enable us to live, work, and relax exactly as we want. When we are organized, our homes, offices, and schedules reflect and encourage who we are, what we want, and where we are going."[1] This begs the question, are the files in the radiology facility organized to provide the staff members with what they want, when they want it?

Records Management: An Overview

Records management involves the systematic control of the creation, maintenance, use, and disposition of records, which include both paper and electronic documents. This process includes the following:

- Setting policies and standards.
- Assigning responsibilities.
- Establishing procedures and guidelines.
- Designing, implementing, and administering systems specifically for managing records.
- Integrating records management into everyday business systems and processes.

Effective records management offers the following benefits:[2]

- Day-to-day operations run smoothly because information needed for decision making and tasks is readily available.
- Staff can deliver services consistently and equitably.
- The rights of employees, patients, and the organization are protected.
- Continuity is ensured in the event of a disaster.

- Records are protected from unauthorized access.
- The facility meets its statutory and regulatory requirements related to archiving, audit, and oversight.
- The organization gains support and protection in litigation.
- Office efficiency and productivity are improved, and documents are retrieved more quickly.
- Organizational and historical data research can be carried out efficiently and accurately.
- Valuable office space is freed up for other purposes and unnecessary purchases of equipment are eliminated, as inactive files are moved to storage and outdated files are destroyed.

Most radiology facilities distinguish between clinical records and nonclinical records. Generally, clinical records include, but are not limited to, patient information, radiology reports, radiology film and electronic images, patient insurance information, radiology or section logbooks, patient charges, examination requests, therapeutic treatment requests, and transcription reports (see Chapter 14). Nonclinical records include personnel files, general business documents, and for facilities that are part of a corporate structure, corporate office documents. These records are the primary focus of this chapter. Financial records are also considered nonclinical records.[3]

Radiology administrators working within a hospital or other large healthcare facility will probably find a records management system in place that includes facility-wide policies and procedures. In a freestanding imaging center, the radiology administrator may have a substantial role in devising, restructuring, and maintaining the records management program. Although professionals trained in records management can be hired (see Box 16.1), either as consultants or staff members, the

---

Box 16.1 Resources for Records Management Training and Professionals

AIIM (Enterprise Content Management Association)
www.aiim.org

American Health Information Management Association (AHIMA)
www.ahima.org

ARMA International (an association for information management professionals)
www.arma.org

Gatlin Education Services
www.gatlineducation.com/recordsmanagement.html

National Archives and Records Administration
www.archives.gov/records-mgmt/training

---

radiology administrator should understand the basics to ensure that the unit's overall needs are met by whatever system is in place.

The three stages of records management are (1) creation and receipt of files, (2) maintenance and use, and (3) disposition.

Creation and Receipt of Files

The personal computer and the Internet have revolutionized the way business is run. Radiology administrators are bombarded daily with e-mails—some of which need only to be read and then deleted, others that require action or response, and still others that need to be referred to on an ongoing basis. To stay on top of the many demands and requests, the radiology administrator must create a filing system for all e-mails. A variety of systems are used, but one of the most commonly accepted approaches is to organize electronic folders by person, project, department (for example, accounting, human resources, information systems, and materials management), vendors, follow-up, and immediate action needed. To maintain system function, e-mails that are no longer needed must be deleted regularly and often. Key messages should be printed out and become part of the paper records system.

The premise for creating paper files, either from e-mail documents or as originals, is easy placement of—and access to—information. There are two basic types of paper files: temporary (working) and permanent (archival). Determining when and how often a file will be used should indicate which type it is.

Working Files

Most new files will be working files and include the following:

- *Action items*—frequently used items requiring regular decisions and action (for example, daily patient volume statistical reports, cost variance reports, and central supply purchase orders).
- *Project items*—plans, notes, and documents related to current projects (for example, capital replacement projects, department renovations or construction, and marketing strategy).
- *Reading items*—must-read materials from any source (for example, trade magazine articles, continuing education material, and equipment updates).
- *Purge items*—outdated material and irrelevant data, often in the form of clutter (for example, outdated trade magazines).

Remember, these working files are temporary files. They will be used, then moved to long-term storage and destroyed at a specified date or when superseded. Use a label maker (a great inexpensive investment), and label folders or boxes as "action," "project," and "reading" files by purpose or function (for example, "Capital Projects" and "Marketing"), or be more specific, such as "ABC Gamma Camera Project." Use broad, generic headings that are meaningful to all users. If the files are shared with supporting assistants or other section supervisors, the categories and headings must make sense to everyone involved (for example, "CT/MRI–Contrast Analysis, 2006").

The headings used will be determined in part by the filing system chosen. An alphabetical system, in which files are arranged alphabetically by the first letter of the heading, is probably the best-known system, but it is not necessarily the most efficient. If the number of files is large, there will probably be duplicate alphabetical file headings, especially with personnel records. The following are other possible filing systems:

- *Subject*—an efficient option if subfolders are used within a folder (for example, "Folder: CAT SCAN–Subfolder: Contrast." However, this option calls for considerable judgment on the part of the person creating the files, and in many cases the subject chosen is open to interpretation.
- *Numerical*—not to be confused with *chronological* order files (see below); reliable for dated material (for example, purchase orders, invoices, bills, dated tasks, and spreadsheets). However, any set of files can be made numerical by assigning sequential numbers to every file, arranging the files numerically, and then creating an index with the number and file content description for easy retrieval. Numerical classification can be applied to any set of records, even if some records are in binders or boxes.
- *Geographical*—appropriate for storage of files from satellite operations, but otherwise of limited usefulness, not the least because so few people have a strong enough geography knowledge to use and maintain the system accurately.
- *Chronological*—a proficient solution for backup files requiring routine review. *Tickler files* are special examples of chronological arrangements; these files are arranged by the day, month, and/or year, indicating the date by which their contents are to be reviewed and/or dealt with.

Here are some additional suggestions to help create a functional filing system:

- Avoid creating "thin" file headings that are hard to keep track of. Use headings that cover a substantial amount of material (up to 2 inches of paper; box containers work well for thicker files).

- Design the system, complete with headings and subheadings, before actually creating the files.
- Use nouns for headings, because adjectives tend to get lost in memory.
- Log or document the filing system for future reference. Create an index of all files, including where each file is located and who has physical possession (called the *custodian*). Create a records inventory, which tracks records series (all documents related to a single process, such as purchase orders, or to a single topic, such as personnel). The records inventory includes who holds the primary copy (copy of record), whether the records are confidential or vital, whether they have historical value, and how long the records should be held. Both the file index and the records inventory should be kept up-to-date (for example, updated when files are added or changes to the system are made). These documents streamline file creation and disposal and ensure that anyone creating new files follows the existing system. Both documents should be created and stored on the facility's computer system, allowing for easy updating and universal access.
- Make it as easy as possible to add new files to the system. Keep a stock of labels, folders (manila and hanging), tabs, and other filing materials close at hand. Always have the label printer ready with new tape. Be ready to quickly create a space for any lost piece of paper.

Archival Files

Archival files are a permanent part of the organization. They include documents related to the incorporation of the facility and other historical benchmarks; key photographs; deeds, architectural drawings, and other items related to physical property; and manuals and reference books. Information contained in archival records may be needed for legal or financial reasons many years after the founding and may be used for annual reports, brochures, or anniversary celebrations. These records should be inventoried for ultimate retrieval, even if they are stored off-site. Box 16.2 shows an example of a radiology department's filing system.

Box 16.2 An Example of a Subject-Alphabetical File System

ADMINISTRATOR BINDERS

(Revised: 6-8-07)

BOOKCASE (Archive)

BUSINESS MANAGEMENT FOR RADIOLOGY
CT 1
CT 2
CT 3

(Continued)

Box 16.2   (Continued)

DIAGNOSTIC ROOMS 1,6, & 8
DIAGNOSTIC ROOM 3
DIAGNOSTIC ROOM 4
DIAGNOSTIC ROOM 5
JCAHO
MANAGEMENT FOR CLINICAL LEADERS
NUCLEAR MEDICINE ROOM 2
OTTO C-ARMS 2005
PET SCANNER
SEQ 2005
STATE HEALTH RULES & REGULATIONS
STRICKEN MEDICAL
VASCULAR ROOM 2
VASCULAR ROOM 3

CABINET ONE (Archival)

BUDGET
POSITION SUMMARY 2006–2007
RESPONSIBILITY STATEMENT 2006

SECRETARY BINDERS (Working)

(Revised: 6-8-07)

BIRTHDAYS
EMPLOYEE SAT SURVEY
EVALUATIONS
GL 290 TRANSACTION REPORT
SAFETY
STOREROOM CATALOG
TB REPORT

FILE CABINET FILES (Archival)

(Revised: 6-8-07)

CAPITAL EQUIPMENT

CAPITAL EQUIPMENT 2007
CAPITAL EQUIPMENT IMAGE CTR
CAPITAL EXPENDITURE REQUEST
CENTRAL AR RAD TX
CHART US ONE
CONSTRUCTION 04
NUCLEAR MEDICINE (Archival)
NUCLEAR MEDICINE CAMERA
PET PATIENT PREP ROOM
PHILIPS 2007 CAPITAL
PURCHASE ORDERS
QUOTES
ROOM 2 CONSTRUCTION
ROOM 2 INSTALLATION
ULTRASOUND (Archival)
VASCULAR (Archival)
VITAL IMAGES
XENON CT

VENDORS (Archival)

VENDOR A
VENDOR B

VENDOR C
VENDOR D
VENDOR E

BI-WEEK/MONTH STATS (Archival)

BI-WEEKLY STATS
MONTHLY STATS

FORMS (Working)

ACCIDENT REPORTS
APPLICATION
ATTENDANCE POLICY
CONSTRUCTION PROJECT REQUEST
COUNSELING RECORD
IN-HOUSE AGENCY
ISR
LEAVE OF ABSENCE REQUEST
LOCKSMITH SERVICES REQUEST
MAINTENANCE WORK ORDER
NEW EMPLOYEE PACKET
OCCURRENCE REPORT
PAYROLL MEMORANDUM
PERSONNEL VACANCY
PRINT SHOP REQUEST
PURCHASE REQUEST
TELECOMMUNICATIONS ORDER REQUEST
TERMINAL EVALUATION
TIMESHEETS
TRANSFER/PROMOTION REQUEST
TRAVEL FORMS
TUITION ASSISTANCE
UNIFORM AUTHORIZATION
WORKERS COMPENSATION

PACS (Archival)

PACS
PACS FACS
PACS JOB DESCRIPTION
PACS MANUAL OF ORGANIZATION
VENDOR M

REPORTS (Working)

ATTENDANCE REPORTING
CT MONTHLY REV VARIANCE
DAILY LATE CHARGES BY CHARGE CODE
EXPENSE DISTRIBUTION DETAIL
EXEPENSE DISTRIBUTION SUMMARY
GL-290
OT REPORT
UNIFORM DEDUCTION

A-Z FILES (Archival)

ABN AUDIT
ACCOUNTING
(ACHE) AMERICAN COLLEGE OF HEALTH CARE EXECUTIVES
ADA

(Continued)

```
ADMINISTRATION
AFTER HOURS PEDS
(AHRA) AMERICAN HEALTH CARE RADIOLOGY ADMINISTRATORS
ARCHITECTS
(ASAP) ADVERTISING SPECIALTIES & PROMOTIONS[
(ASRT) AR SOCIETY OF RADIOLGIC TECHNOLOGIST
CORPORATE COMPLIANCE
CPT CODE
CRITICAL TESTS
(DEA) DRUG ENFORCEMENT ASSOCIATION
DEPARTMENT HEADS
DEPARTMENT OF HEALTH
DISASTER COMMUNICATION
DISASTER SHEET
DOCTORS CREDENTIALS
(EAP) EMPLOYEE ASSISTANCE PROGRAM
EMPLOYEE OF THE MONTH
EMPLOYEE SATISFACTION
EMPLOYEE WELLNESS HANDBOOK
FIT TEAM
FMLA
(GAO) GOVERNMENT ACCOUNTABILITY OFFICE
GRANT REQUESTS
HIPPA
HMI MNGT
HUMAN RESOURCES
INFECTIOUS CONTROL
INJURY REPORTS
INPATIENT SATISFACTION
(IS) INFORMATION SYSTEMS
JCAHO
JRCERT
LEAVE OF ABSENCE
MAINTENANCE
MANAGEMENT SYSTEMS
MARKETING
MATERIALS MANAGEMENT
NURSES
OSHA
OUTPATIENT SATISFACTION
PATIENT CARE COMPLIANCE FORUM
PATIENT IDENTIFICATION
QUALITY ASSURANCE
RADIATION SAFETY
RADIOLOGISTS
RIS
RN/LPN
SAFETY COMMITTEE
(SCAR) SOCIETY FOR COMPUTER APPLICATIONS IN RADIOLOGY
SENTINEL EVENT
STROKE
SUPPLY CHAIN–HOEHN
SURVEY COMPLAINTS
TAX EXEMPT NUMBER
TELECOM
TELECOMMUTING
TOASTMASTERS–YACOBACK
TRAX-FOX
TWENTY-FOUR/SEVEN
UNAPPROVED INVOICES
VENDOR HEALTHCARE
VHA GROUPING
VITAL STATISTICS
WASTE MANAGEMENT
WORK INJURIES
```

SECRETARY FILES (Working)

(Revised: 6-8-07)

ACTIVE EMPLOYEE LIST
DISCIPLINARY ACTION
DRUG FORMULARY
EVALUATION INFORMATION
FAX COVER SHEETS
FILM LIBRARY REPORTS
INVOICE COPIES
LETTERS/MEMOS
LPN/RN EVALUATIONS
MENUS
NET LEARNING
OCCUPATIONAL EXPOSURE RECORD
PERSONNEL FILE CHECKLIST
PHYSICAL INVENTORY
PTO HOURS TAKEN
RADIATION DOSIMETRY REPORT
RADIATION EXPOSURE HISTORY
SERVICE AWARDS
STOREROOM CATALOG
TIMECARDS
VOICEMAIL TRAINING GUIDE

Maintenance and Use of Files

File Locations and Storage Fixtures

Unlike radiology images, organization files do not have a direct impact on patient care and most likely will not contribute to revenues. If floor space is limited, storage of these files will be a significant issue. According to records management consultant Gloria Gold, 85% of all records will never be looked at once they are filed. Of the remaining 15% that will be used, 98% of use occurs within the first year of filing.[4] To increase the likelihood of usefulness, working files need to be accessible. Decide who will be using the files, when they will be used, and how much room is available for storage. Should the files be in or close to an individual desk for frequent retrieval? Or should they be centrally located, so they are accessible to several people? Can they be stored off-site? Is security a factor? If so, how will security be ensured—for example, with storage in a locked room or locked cabinet—and who must have access?

File cabinets can be vertical, lateral, or open shelf. Wall storage units and rolling file racks are good choices. The type of organizing fixture depends on space and needs. Binders work well for storing articles, newspaper clippings, reports, job descriptions, policies and procedures, and other reference materials. If it is necessary to hang on to purposeful dated material, such as trade magazines or books, cardboard boxes will suffice. For confidential records, a locked file cabinet, lockable desk

---

drawer, or closet with a key lock may be adequate to keep them secure, but only if the storage space is kept locked and access to the key or combination is strictly limited (see Box 16.3).

Box 16.3 Information Sensitivity Policy

1.0 Purpose

The Information Sensitivity Policy is intended to help employees determine what information can be disclosed to non-employees, as well as the relative sensitivity of information that should not be disclosed outside of the organization without proper authorization.

The information covered in these guidelines includes, but is not limited to, information that is either stored or shared via any means. This includes: electronic information, information on paper, and information shared orally or visually (such as telephone and video conferencing).

All employees should familiarize themselves with the information labeling and handling guidelines that follow this introduction. It should be noted that the sensitivity level definitions were created as guidelines and to emphasize common sense steps that you can take to protect <Company Name> Confidential information (e.g., <Company Name> Confidential information should not be left unattended in conference rooms).

Please Note: The impact of these guidelines on daily activity should be minimal. Questions about the proper classification of a specific piece of information should be addressed to your manager. Questions about these guidelines should be addressed to Infosec.

2.0 Scope

All <Company Name> information is categorized into two main classifications:

- <Company Name> Public
- <Company Name> Confidential

<Company Name> Public information is information that has been declared public knowledge by someone with the authority to do so, and can freely be given to anyone without any possible damage to <Company Name> Systems, Inc.

<Company Name> Confidential contains all other information. It is a continuum, in that it is understood that some information is more sensitive than other information, and should be protected in a more secure manner. Included is information that should be protected very closely, such as trade secrets, development programs, potential acquisition targets, and other information integral to the success of our company. Also included in <Company Name> Confidential is information that is less critical, such as telephone directories, general corporate information, personnel information, etc., which does not require as stringent a degree of protection.

A subset of <Company Name> Confidential information is "<Company Name> Third Party Confidential" information. This is confidential information belonging or pertaining to another corporation which has been entrusted to <Company Name> by that company under non-disclosure agreements and other contracts. Examples of this type of information include everything from joint development efforts to vendor lists, customer orders, and supplier information. Information in this category ranges from extremely sensitive to information about the fact that we've connected a supplier/vendor into <Company Name>'s network to support our operations.

<Company Name> personnel are encouraged to use common sense judgment in securing <Company Name> Confidential information to the proper extent. If an employee is uncertain of the sensitivity of a particular piece of information, he/she should contact their manager

3.0 Policy

The Sensitivity Guidelines below provides details on how to protect information at varying sensitivity levels. Use these guidelines as a reference only, as <Company Name> Confidential information in each

---

Box 16.3   (Continued)

column may necessitate more or less stringent measures of protection depending upon the circumstances and the nature of the <Company Name> Confidential information in question.

3.1 Minimal Sensitivity: General corporate information; some personnel and technical information
Marking guidelines for information in hardcopy or electronic form.

Note: any of these markings may be used with the additional annotation of "3rd Party Confidential."

Marking is at the discretion of the owner or custodian of the information. If marking is desired, the words "<Company Name> Confidential" may be written or designated in a conspicuous place on or in the information in question. Other labels that may be used include "<Company Name> Proprietary" or similar labels at the discretion of your individual business unit or department. Even if no marking is present, <Company Name> information is presumed to be "<Company Name> Confidential" unless expressly determined to be <Company Name> Public information by a <Company Name> employee with authority to do so.

Access: <Company Name> employees, contractors, people with a business need to know.

Distribution within <Company Name>: Standard interoffice mail, approved electronic mail and electronic file transmission methods.

Distribution outside of <Company Name> internal mail: U.S. mail and other public or private carriers, approved electronic mail and electronic file transmission methods.

Electronic distribution: No restrictions except that it be sent to only approved recipients.

Storage: Keep from view of unauthorized people; erase whiteboards, do not leave in view on table-top. Machines should be administered with security in mind. Protect from loss; electronic information should have individual access controls where possible and appropriate.

Disposal/Destruction: Deposit outdated paper information in specially marked disposal bins on <Company Name> premises; electronic data should be expunged/cleared. Reliably erase or physically destroy media.

Penalty for deliberate or inadvertent disclosure: Up to and including termination, possible civil and/or criminal prosecution to the full extent of the law.

3.2 More Sensitive: Business, financial, technical, and most personnel information

Marking guidelines for information in hardcopy or electronic form.

Note: any of these markings may be used with the additional annotation of "3rd Party Confidential." As the sensitivity level of the information increases, you may, in addition or instead of marking the information "<Company Name> Confidential" or "<Company Name> Proprietary," wish to label the information "<Company Name> Internal Use Only" or other similar labels at the discretion of your individual business unit or department to denote a more sensitive level of information. However, marking is discretionary at all times.

Access: <Company Name> employees and non-employees with signed non-disclosure agreements who have a business need to know.

Distribution within <Company Name>: Standard interoffice mail, approved electronic mail and electronic file transmission methods.

Distribution outside of <Company Name> internal mail: Sent via U.S. mail or approved private carriers.

Electronic distribution: No restrictions to approved recipients within <Company Name>, but should be encrypted or sent via a private link to approved recipients outside of <Company Name> premises.

Storage: Individual access controls are highly recommended for electronic information.

Disposal/Destruction: In specially marked disposal bins on <Company Name> premises; electronic data should be expunged/cleared. Reliably erase or physically destroy media.

Penalty for deliberate or inadvertent disclosure: Up to and including termination, possible civil and/or criminal prosecution to the full extent of the law.

3.3 Most Sensitive: Trade secrets & marketing, operational, personnel, financial, source code, & technical information integral to the success of our company

(Continued)

Box 16.3   (Continued)

Marking guidelines for information in hardcopy or electronic form.

Note: any of these markings may be used with the additional annotation of "3rd Party Confidential." To indicate that <Company Name> Confidential information is very sensitive, you may should label the information "<Company Name> Internal: Registered and Restricted," "<Company Name> Eyes Only," "<Company Name> Confidential" or similar labels at the discretion of your individual business unit or department. Once again, this type of <Company Name> Confidential information need not be marked, but users should be aware that this information is very sensitive and be protected as such.

Access: Only those individuals (<Company Name> employees and non-employees) designated with approved access and signed non-disclosure agreements.

Distribution within <Company Name>: Delivered direct—signature required, envelopes stamped confidential, or approved electronic file transmission methods.

Distribution outside of <Company Name> internal mail: Delivered direct; signature required; approved private carriers.

Electronic distribution: No restrictions to approved recipients within <Company Name>, but it is highly recommended that all information be strongly encrypted.

Storage: Individual access controls are very highly recommended for electronic information. Physical security is generally used, and information should be stored in a physically secured computer.

Disposal/Destruction: Strongly Encouraged: In specially marked disposal bins on <Company Name> premises; electronic data should be expunged/cleared. Reliably erase or physically destroy media.

Penalty for deliberate or inadvertent disclosure: Up to and including termination, possible civil and/or criminal prosecution to the full extent of the law.

4.0 Enforcement

Any employee found to have violated this policy may be subject to disciplinary action, up to and including termination of employment.

5.0 Definitions

Terms and Definitions

Appropriate measures

To minimize risk to <Company Name> from an outside business connection. <Company Name> computer use by competitors and unauthorized personnel must be restricted so that, in the event of an attempt to access <Company Name> corporate information, the amount of information at risk is minimized.

Configuration of <Company Name>-to-other business connections

Connections shall be set up to allow other businesses to see only what they need to see. This involves setting up both applications and network configurations to allow access to only what is necessary.

Delivered Direct; Signature Required

Do not leave in interoffice mail slot, call the mail room for special pick-up of mail.

Approved Electronic File Transmission Methods

Includes supported FTP clients and Web browsers.

Envelopes Stamped Confidential

You are not required to use a special envelope. Put your document(s) into an interoffice envelope, seal it, address it, and stamp it confidential.

Approved Electronic Mail

Includes all mail systems supported by the IT Support Team. These include, but are not necessarily limited to, [insert corporate supported mailers here …]. If you have a business need to use other mailers contact the appropriate support organization.

Box 16.3   (Continued)

Approved Encrypted email and files

Techniques include the use of DES and PGP. DES encryption is available via many different public domain packages on all platforms. PGP use within <Company Name> is done via a license. Please contact the appropriate support organization if you require a license.

Company Information System Resources

Company Information System Resources include, but are not limited to, all computers, their data and programs, as well as all paper information and any information at the Internal Use Only level and above.

Expunge

To reliably erase or expunge data on a PC or Mac you must use a separate program to overwrite data, supplied as a part of Norton Utilities. Otherwise, the PC or Mac's normal erasure routine keeps the data intact until overwritten. The same thing happens on UNIX machines, but data is much more difficult to retrieve on UNIX systems.

Individual Access Controls

Individual Access Controls are methods of electronically protecting files from being accessed by people other than those specifically designated by the owner. On UNIX machines, this is accomplished by careful use of the chmod command (use *man chmod* to find out more about it). On Mac's and PC's, this includes using passwords on screensavers, such as Disklock.

Insecure Internet Links

Insecure Internet Links are all network links that originate from a locale or travel over lines that are not totally under the control of <Company Name>.

Encryption

Secure <Company Name> Sensitive information in accordance with the *Acceptable Encryption Policy*. International issues regarding encryption are complex. Follow corporate guidelines on export controls on cryptography, and consult your manager and/or corporate legal services for further guidance.

One Time Password Authentication

One Time Password Authentication on Internet connections is accomplished by using a one time password token to connect to <Company Name>'s internal network over the Internet. Contact your support organization for more information on how to set this up.

Physical Security

Physical security means either having actual possession of a computer at all times, or locking the computer in an unusable state to an object that is immovable. Methods of accomplishing this include having a special key to unlock the computer so it can be used, thereby ensuring that the computer cannot be simply rebooted to get around the protection. If it is a laptop or other portable computer, never leave it alone in a conference room, hotel room or on an airplane seat, etc. Make arrangements to lock the device in a hotel safe, or take it with you. In the office, always use a lockdown cable. When leaving the office for the day, secure the laptop and any other sensitive material in a locked drawer or cabinet.

Private Link

A Private Link is an electronic communications path that <Company Name> has control over its entire distance. For example, all <Company Name> networks are connected via a private link. A computer with modem connected via a standard land line (not cell phone) to another computer has established a private link. ISDN lines to employees' homes are a private link. <Company Name> also has established private links to other companies, so that all email correspondence can be sent in a more secure manner. Companies which <Company Name> has established private links include all announced acquisitions and some short-term temporary links

6.0 Revision History

Source: Reference material from http://www.sans.org/resources/policies/Information_Sensitivity_Policy. pdf. Accessed November 22, 2006. Used with permission from The SANS Institute

True working files are frequently taken out of cabinets, of course, and may spend more time outside of storage than inside. The best filing system will soon disintegrate into chaos if files are left to pile up on desks and office floors, given to staff members in other units, or removed from the building. If the facility's imaging library has a sign-out system, consider adapting it to the organization files. Facilities with many records may want to invest in barcoding or radiofrequency identification technology (commonly used by package carriers). These techniques electronically track the movement of records from office to office or even out of the office and allow for periodic auditing of records.

For files in current use, invest in appropriate desktop or wall-mounted fixtures, such as multilevel, slotted, cascading, or stackable trays. "Hot files" are receptacles that attach to the wall or the side of a desk and hold approximately 100 sheets of paper. Multiple hot files can be categorized (for example, "Mail," "Journals/Magazines," "Hospital Reports," "For Review," "To Be Signed," and "Other").

Product samples, sample radiographic film, photographs, and catalogs are examples of items that may not readily fit into file folders but do need to be retained and retrieved. Possible solutions for filing or storing such items include the following:

- Boxes that hold both samples and hanging file folders.
- Cardboard, metal, or plastic holders (great for filing magazines and catalogs) that sit on a shelf.
- Tubes that accommodate large, rolled-up prints or renovation/architectural plans.
- Large envelopes that hold oversized papers in the bottom of a file drawer or box.
- Plastic sleeves that go into binders and are suitable for photographs, small brochures, and catalogs.

Special Categories of Records

Personnel Records—The role of effective documentation in the management of human resources is to provide the ability to reference an employee's personnel data when required by the radiology administrator or senior management. Managing and maintaining the radiology facility's human resources can be a challenging and difficult administrative function. Fortunately, with today's highly sophisticated hardware (specifically, the office PC) and software, many of the time-consuming tasks of manual paperwork filing and calendar or statistical manipulation have become obsolete.

Personnel records management is readily accepted as a management function. Operating the business systems of information control, while analyzing and interpreting the dynamic statistics of human asset evaluation, allows the radiology administrator to make rational management decisions. These decisions encompass areas such as effective labor planning, project planning, strategic planning, workflow analysis, and overall best practices to use the department's human technical resources for daily operational radiologic services.

The radiology facility's personnel records represent not only information on individual and overall labor resources but also on the history of the facility's operations. These records provide quick and easy access to the individual employee's relevant data, including address, telephone number, date of birth, identification number, hire date, pay rate, pay range, and performance evaluation date.

Most healthcare organizations maintain an *official* personnel file (copy of record) in the human resources department, whose role in effective documentation is to ensure the continuity of personnel record management storage. The radiology administrator and human resources administrator should devise guidelines outlining which records will be documented and stored in the official human resources file, based on legal and organizational criteria. In some instances, duplicate documents or records will need to be stored in the radiology facility's administrative offices. These replicated records can be referred to as *working files*.

The personnel record comprises both paper and electronic documents, regardless of their location, including the documents in an official file as well as a working file. A personnel file should be created for each employee and should include the job application, letters of reference, background check reports, and other documentation related to hiring; job performance documents, such as current job description, performance evaluations, counseling records, verbal and written warnings, and letters of commendation; documentation of professional accomplishments and continuing education; and copies of license certifications and renewals. (A copy of the license/certification is no longer adequate for facility accreditation by The Joint Commission; evidence of confirmation of license renewal must be provided.) Subfolders can assist in eliminating multiple searches for documents—for example, "(a) employee (folder): Doe, John A.; (b) (subfolder): License/Continuing Education." Personnel records are confidential and should be stored in a secure manner, as described above.

General Business Records—In a large, multidepartment organization such as a hospital, the radiology department often maintains duplicate working files of relevant general business and corporate office records, whereas the originals (copies of record) are kept with the originating corporate department or main general business department. These records include documents related to purchasing, materials management, accounting and finance, and administration, and they range from internal memorandums and electronic communications (e-mail) to purchase orders. Stand-alone facilities may find that only one set of records, accessible to both the radiology administrator and nonclinical managers, is necessary.

Capital Equipment Purchase and Maintenance Records—Record keeping for capital equipment purchases is necessary for the radiology administrator to have a good understanding of how, when, and why the equipment was purchased and how the purchase agreement was worded. Any of several different filing systems may be used, as described above; a commonly used method for capital equipment management is to create a separate folder or binder on each piece of capital equipment purchased. Identifying the capital equipment by year of purchase, vendor name, or equipment title will allow for the retrieval of relevant and pertinent information in one place that is easily accessible to the radiology administrator when needed.

The PC is useful in many aspects of records management and is particularly valuable to maintain selected capital equipment maintenance records. The same separate folder or binder process used in a paper environment can be duplicated on a PC, with a separate subfolder for each piece of equipment. Files can be organized by fiscal year or calendar date, vendor-specific name, or equipment type. All preventive maintenance and repairs should be logged in this document. Doing so ensures that all pertinent information regarding the equipment is located in one place when the radiology administrator needs immediate access to the document during inspections.

Vital Records—Each of the three previous sets of records contains a subset, the vital records. Vital records are records that are essential to the facility's operation; should a natural or man-made disaster occur, having these records will make business recovery faster and more efficient (see the Sidebar). The types of records that may be vital include incorporation documents, payroll records, insurance policies, inventory lists, supplier lists, and contracts. Vital records require special handling. They can be duplicated or put onto microfilm and stored in a safe, yet accessible place away from the facility and perhaps even in another state, or they can be stored in an onsite vault or fire-rated file cabinet.

SIDEBAR: A Records Recovery Plan

Emergency response and disaster preparedness have a long tradition in healthcare organizations, and most facilities have a detailed disaster plan in place. However, any existing plan should be reviewed to evaluate its effectiveness with regard to the organization's vital records. According to the National Archives and Records Administration, the federal agency responsible for protecting priceless documents such as the US Constitution, a facility's disaster plan should include records recovery, with details on the following steps:

1. Notify the appropriate individuals immediately to provide details about the nature of the emergency and the level of threat to the records.

2. Assess the damage to records as soon as possible after the emergency, keeping in mind that records in different formats (for example, microfilm versus paper) may suffer varying degrees of damage.

3. Take steps to stabilize the records to prevent further damage, assembling a predesignated team to accomplish this step in the event of a major disaster (confidential records can be handled only by authorized personnel). Separate undamaged records from damaged ones wherever possible to eliminate additional damage and speed recovery.

4. Consult with vendors that provide record recovery services, based on the assessment. The plan should include a list of specialists with area of expertise and contact information. Because these vendors tend to be highly specialized (for example, only working with water-damaged paper records recovery), the list should include a full range of vendors to allow for all the potential risks.

5. Recover the records, or provide replacements for nonrecoverable documents.

Because water, fire, and smoke have the greatest potential to damage records, the National Archives suggests having basic supplies accessible to deal with these risks. Items include sponges, plastic storage bags, plastic crates (for safely moving quantities of wet documents), and a wet/dry vacuum. The full list can be found at http://www.archives.gov/records-mgmt/vital-records/appendix-d.html#PartXI.

Source: National Archives and Records Administration. Available at: http://www.archives.gov/records-mgmt/vital-records/index.html. Accessed March 16, 2007.

Record Disposition

After the project is finished or the action is completed, a decision must be made on whether to discard the file or move it into the permanent file category. Many files will be moved to the permanent category, but some files (for example, a file that contains only duplicates of records filed elsewhere) do not need to be retained. It is also advisable to review items within a file before moving it, as some items, such as personal notes, may be eliminated. Decide if the items contain quality information worth keeping and storing. Are the items timely? Can they be obtained elsewhere? Are they accurate and reliable (and will they continue to be so)? How will they be used in the future?

Before files are stored, they should be assigned a disposition date based on a retention schedule. This document specifies how long records are kept before disposition. Without a retention schedule, office files would eventually flow into all available space and make finding and accessing records inefficient. The criteria on which to base a retention schedule follow:[4]

- *Legal needs.* Statutes, codes of federal regulations, and accrediting body mandates set timeframes for the retention of many records. Table 16.1 provides guidelines for the retention of nonclinical files. However, because of state and local variations and changes in regulations over time, before assigning a disposition date the radiology administrator should consult the human resources or corporate compliance department and review the latest regulations for the ACR, The Joint

Table 16.1 Guidelines for Record Destruction*

Department	Name of Record	Destroy Date
Accounting	Responsibility reports Budget Payroll and time/attendance records Paid invoices Cash receipts/deposit records Audits	10 years 7 years 7 years 5 years 4 years 10 years
Materials management	Requests for purchase Purchase orders Bids Purchasing contracts	13th month 13th month 13th month 1 year after expiration
Human resources	Job descriptions Policies (current and official) Absentee reports Accident reports Criminal background checks OIG/GSA screens Applications Personnel files Employee schedules	When job description revised Maintained until revised 3 years 3 years 4 years after termination 4 years after termination 1 year 2 years after termination (terminal evaluations, written warnings, and hiring documents are kept permanently) 1 year
Corporate office	Staff meeting minutes Competency records Organizational charts Contracts General correspondence HIPAA-related audits or reviews	3 years 5 years 1 year 1 year after expiration date Current year and prior 3 years (hard copy and e-mail) 6 years

*OIG indicates Office of the Inspector General; GSA, General Services Administration; HIPAA, Health Insurance Portability and Accountability Act.

Commission, and the American Hospital Association, as well as local or state laws such as the MQSA.

- *Administrative and fiscal needs.* These needs are set by the facility itself; they cannot be less than the legal needs, but they may be more. For example, business correspondence of a facility's partners and senior staff might be retained longer than the correspondence of lower management.
- *Need for disaster protection for vital records.* If records are determined to be vital to the facility's function, they need to be protected in the event of a natural or man-made disaster. Many vital records are superseded by subsequent documents; for example, each pay period creates a current set of vital records, which supersedes the previous records. The retention schedule should take into account which records should be designated vital, how often they are updated and outdated copies are destroyed, and how the records (or copies) will be protected.
- *Archive needs.* As has been noted, archival files are a permanent part of the organization. They include documents related to incorporation of the facility and other historical benchmarks; key photographs; and deeds, architectural drawings, and other items related to physical property and capital equipment. Information contained in archival records may be needed for legal or financial reasons many years after the facility's founding and may be used for annual reports, brochures, or anniversary celebrations. These records should be handled in much the same manner as vital records.

Maintain the retention schedule separately from the files themselves. The dates for review and disposition should show up on a calendar (or a shared calendar) and should be the same every year so that the process becomes part of the facility's routine. With a detailed retention schedule, most files can be disposed of by support staff, with minimal oversight by the radiology administrator or the record's custodian.

Record Destruction Process

By referring to the retention schedule, staff members can cull paper records that are ready for disposal relatively quickly. Some records may need evaluation by the administrator or record custodian (for example, files previously designated as archival that now appear to be outdated). If some records have been stored in boxes without adequate identification, one person can refer to the retention schedule as another pulls files for review. Files that are designated to be destroyed can be put to one side until they are noted in the record inventory as destroyed. No file should be destroyed before the inventory has been updated.

Confidential records should be handled only by authorized staff. They should be shredded only after the destruction has been noted on the record inventory.

For electronic records, the procedure is much more complicated. Data will have been frequently backed up onto hard drives, CD-ROMs, or other removable media. Network data are backed up frequently—often hourly, daily, weekly, and monthly. Information is archived continuously, and frequently at a redundant, remote location. Thus, information exists in multiple locations. A typical corporate e-mail could exist in as many as half a dozen places: the sender's laptop (in three or four places), the outbound mail server, the backup of that server, the inbound mail server, the recipient's computer, any carbon copies (CCs), and of course, any potential printouts. Furthermore, add telecommuters—such as transcriptionists, staff members working from their home computers, and staff members using USB thumb drive storage and other portable hard drives such as iPods—and the logistical nightmare with regard to destroying any given electronic file becomes obvious.

Security professionals in the organization's information systems department should automate the process of e-file document destruction based on the retention schedule. Doing so will ensure that the deletion includes all the many places where the document may exist and will prevent documents from being overlooked, forgotten, or not being deleted properly.

The Value of Document Destruction Policies

Records management experts estimate that 30% of all records in an office and 40% of records in storage can and should be destroyed.[4] Storage is expensive and often consumes potential revenue-producing space (that is, the film library). Furthermore, no purpose is served in keeping documents that are no longer useful for daily business operations. Because of the inability to quickly retrieve paper documents, obsolete records represent only a cost to the healthcare organization.

In the electronic world, of course, storage costs are much lower. Indeed, to a great extent, it may be more expensive to delete documents effectively than simply to retain them. The backups have already been made in the ordinary course of business. To delete documents, a staff member would have to remount the backup media, examine the files, determine which ones are needed and which ones are no longer needed, and effectively delete the files that are no longer needed. The records that may be needed are archived, and the process is repeated periodically. In addition, because the documents are stored in multiple locations, this process would have to be repeated on multiple backups, desktops, and laptops to ensure the deletion of a document. If a document is only partially deleted, it must still be produced in discovery for litigation, but the cost of compliance has greatly increased. Generally, it is much cheaper to just store the documents.

So why have a destruction policy for electronic records? The main reason for healthcare organizations to establish a document destruction policy, including the destruction of electronic records, is to protect the organization from undue litigation. Someone is going to want the records—perhaps a disgruntled former employee, an injured vendor or patient, a competitor, a regulator, or a prosecutor. Modern litigation is the art of discovery, which means making the other side bring out its records. The more records that are available, the greater the expense in locating them and the more information that is potentially useful in litigation. Thus, a typical corporate document destruction policy might specify that any document that is not required to be kept by law or needed for the ongoing business of the healthcare organization is to be deleted 24 hours after it is created. However, should litigation occur and it is known that particular documents or categories of documents may be relevant, the document destruction policy should be suspended. The organization's legal counsel can assist with the next step of conveying transfer of approved documents to the requesting parties.

The radiology administrator, in consultation with other record custodians and senior management, should establish a clear and reasonable destruction policy. The radiology facility's policy should ensure that this policy is applied to active and archived documents equally, and to both paper and electronic documents.

Written Procedures: Ensuring System Maintenance

Each of the processes described in this chapter should be written into a records management policy and procedures manual that covers both on-site storage and files stored off site (see Chapter 14). By providing procedures that have been well thought out, the radiology administrator helps ensure that staff members create new files that conform to the system, that new staff members can be trained to use the system, and that records maintenance becomes routine.

The procedures should spell out each step in sequence and specify who (by title) is responsible. If dates are relevant, they should be provided, as should the names of any forms to be used. The manual can be retained electronically, with a master paper copy available in key administrative areas and at any off-site storage facilities.

Conclusion

The continuous balance of time, space, and insight in the management of documents is a challenge, but the organization of information is critical to the effective operation of any healthcare facility. Efficiency and productivity result when the necessary information is available when and where it is wanted. Modern records management has been professionalized and has much to offer radiology administrators and other managers who must oversee organization files.

References

1. Morgenstern J. *Organizing from the Inside Out*. New York, NY: Henry Holt and Co; 1998.

2. National Archives and Records Administration. Records managers. Frequently asked questions about records management in general. Available at: http://www. archives. gov/records-mgmt/faqs/general.html. Accessed November 20, 2006.

3. Sferrella SM, Allen ML, Reitter MS, eds. *Financial Management in Radiology*. Sudbury, MA: American Healthcare Radiology Administrators; 2004.

4. Gold G. *How to Set Up and Implement a Records Management System*. New York, NY: American Management Association, AMACOM; 1995.

Index

Payback period (PBP) analysis, 191, 192*s*
Peer review, 25–26, 63
Philanthropy, 70–72
Physician peer-review programs, 25–26
Plan Do Check Act (PDCA) Method, 49–50,
    50*b*
Plan Do Study Act (PDSA) Method, 57–58
Policy and procedure manuals, 133–136,
    137*b*, 279
Press kit, 161
Print communications, 129–131, 131*s*
Privacy Rule, 227–228, 228*s*, 229, 229*b*
Procedure volume, 4
Processes
    defined, 47
    prioritizing, 48
    quality control monitoring of, 47, 47*s*, 48–50,
        50*b*, 51, 51*b*
    types of, 48–49
PROCESS method, 51, 51*b*
Productivity
    characteristics of, 18
    management of, 18–19
    peaks and valleys in, 20, 20*f*, 21*f*
Profit margin, 68
Pro forma documents, 69, 69*b*, 70
Protected health information (PHI), 177
Public relations, 151, 157–158

Q

Quality assurance, 45
    in compliance processes, 31
    goals of, 31–32
    scheduled meetings on, 32
Quality control, 42
Quality improvement (QI)
    associated with accreditation, 24
    balanced scorecards in, 113–115, 119
    basics of, 41–43, 43*s*–45*s*
    communicating achievements of, 113, 114,
        119–120, 121, 121*s*, 122–123, 124*f*
    data collection in, 59–62
    departmental dashboards of, 120–121,
        121*b*, 122
    goals of, 113, 114, 119–120, 121, 121*s*,
        122, 124*f*
    measurement tools for, 51–52, 52*f*, 53, 53*f*, 54,
        54*f*, 55, 55*f*, 56
    monitoring processes in, 47, 47*s*, 48–50, 50*b*,
        51, 51*b*
    Nine Dimensions of Performance in, 46, 46*s*,
        47, 47*s*, 48–50, 50*b*, 51, 51*b*
    organizations/agencies practicing, 62–63, 64*t*

Pareto charts in, 51–52, 52*f*, 53
    performance measures and indicators in, 46,
        46*s*, 47, 47*s*, 48–50, 50*b*, 51, 51*b*
    Plan Do Check Act (PDCA) Method of,
        49–50, 50*b*
    practices and initiatives of, 57–59
    procedural, 122, 124*f*
    PROCESS method of, 51, 51*b*
    resources/accrediting bodies and regulations
        of, 25, 62–63, 64*t*
    root cause analysis method in, 56–57
    staff empowerment and, 63, 65–66
Quality management, 42
Quality planning, 42

R

Radiologist meetings, 172–173
Radiology information system (RIS), 141
    connectivity with modalities, 6
    technology applications in, 184–185, 190
    value-driven approach to, 195–221
RADPEER, 25, 26
Raising Capital (Sherman), 73
Rate of return (ROR) analysis, 191, 192*s*, 193
Recognized Continuing Education Evaluation
    Mechanism (RCEEM), 173
Records management, 259–280
    barcoding/radiofrequency identification of,
        272
    capital equipment purchase/maintenance
        records in, 274
    categories of, 272–274
    clinical and nonclinical records in, 260
    creation and receipt of files, 261–263,
        263*b*–267*b*
    destruction policies/schedules for, 277–279
    disposition of, 275–276, 276*t*, 277–279
    emergency/disaster recovery plan for, 275*s*
    filing systems for, 263–264, 264*b*–267*b*
    general business records in, 273–274
    information sensitivity policies of, 268*b*–271*b*
    maintenance and use of files in, 267–268,
        268*b*–271*b*, 272
    permanent (archival) records in, 261, 263
    personnel records in, 272–273
    process and benefits of, 259–260
    resources for, 260*b*
    vital records in, 274
    working files (temporary) in, 261–262
Redundancy, 235–237, 251–252
Redundant array of inexpensive disks (RAID),
    236
Referral levels, 4